Kirby I. Bland • Michael G. Sarr
Markus W. Büchler • Attila Csendes
Oliver James Garden • John Wong
(Editors)

# Surgery of the Esophagus and Stomach

## Handbooks in General Surgery

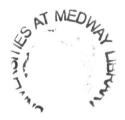

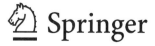

Springer

*Editors*

Kirby I. Bland
University of Alabama
Birmingham
Department of Surgery
Birmingham Alabama
USA

Attila Csendes
University of Chile
Clinical Hospital
Department of Surgery
Santiago
Chile

Michael G. Sarr
Mayo Clinic
Division of Gastroenterologic &
General Surgery
Rochester Minnesota
USA

Oliver James Garden
University of Edinburgh
Royal Infirmary
Department of Surgery
Edinburgh
United Kingdom

Markus W. Büchler
Universitätsklinikum Heidelberg
Chirurgische Klinik
Abt. Allgemeine, Viszerale und
Unfallchirurgie
Heidelberg
Germany

John Wong
Queen Mary Hospital
Department of Surgery
Hong Kong

ISBN 978-1-84996-437-1        e-ISBN 978-1-84996-438-8
DOI 10.1007/978-1-84996-438-8
Springer London Dordrecht Heidelberg New York

British Library Cataloguing in Publication Data
A catalogue record for this book is available from the British Library

Library of Congress Control Number: 2010937963

*Cover design:* eStudioCalamar Figueres/Berlin

Printed on acid-free paper

Springer is part of Springer Science+Business Media (www.springer.com)

# Preface

The editors designed the original textbook, *General Surgery: Principles and International Practice*, from which this shorter paperback monograph on surgery of the esophagus and stomach was taken to be an accessible, concise, and state-of-the-art volume that explores and documents evolutionary principles in the practice of surgery. This work is aimed at the general surgeon and the resident in training. The scientific community continues to witness extraordinary advances in the therapy of both benign and malignant surgical diseases of various organ sites. Much of this progress has been evident over the past decade with new concepts and techniques of management that allow the surgeon to integrate this discipline with medicine, pharmacology, immunology, biostatistics, pathology, genetics, medical and radiation oncology, and diagnostic radiology and imaging. Further, each of these major disciplines contributes a small component for the diagnostic and therapeutic approaches to clinical care; hence the comprehensive planning, integration, and provision of patient care throughout the preoperative, intraoperative, and postoperative phases of care remains essential in the successful practice of our specialty.

The editors acknowledge that the aim of this work is to provide an illustrative, instructive, and comprehensive review that depicts the rationale of basic operative principles essential to surgical therapy. In organizing this monograph, the editors chose authors renowned in the disciplines for illustrating, forming, and depicting in a comprehensive fashion the surgical therapy expectant for metabolic, infectious, endocrine, and neoplastic abnormalities in adult and pediatric patients **from a truly international and multi-continental perspective**. The editors and authors were chosen carefully from across geographies and also from multi-cultural and diverse locations. While the authors consider this text to be inclusive regarding the technical and operative conditions for perioperative care in this field, its purpose should not be intended to replace standard textbooks of surgery nor should it be considered complete in its coverage of pathophysiologic disorders. In contrast, this monograph is organized to familiarize practicing surgeons, residents, and fellows with state-of-the-art surgical principles and techniques essential to contemporary practice. Therefore, the tenor of this monograph on surgery of the esophagus and stomach has been developed to coexist with other major surgical reference texts that are dedicated—some in more comprehensive fashion—to the therapy of individual organs of systemic diseases. This monograph is much more a "working text" for the practicing surgeon with emphasis on diagnosis and treatment of esophagus and stomach disorders. Along with this monograph, nine other paperback monographs are available and focus on the general principles of surgery, trauma, critical care, small bowel, colorectal, liver and biliary, pancreas and spleen, oncology, and endocrine organs all adapted from the primary textbook—*General Surgery: Principles and International Practice*.

The chapters in this monograph on surgery of the esophagus and stomach include a condensed bibliography of highly selective journal articles, reviews, and text. In this manner of attempting to be concise, we hope to provide a precise focus for the education of the reader relative to accepted surgical principles involved in patient care. Moreover, the editors have sought to provide a counterpoint view for the selection of therapy by presenting at the opening of each chapter a list of "Pearls and Pitfalls" that highlight particular concerns or controversies. The chapters provide pertinent, though not exhaustive, summaries of anatomy and physiology, a history of surgical illness, and stages of operative approaches with relevant technical considerations outlined in an easily understandable manner. Complications are reviewed when appropriate for the organ system, diseases, and problem. The text is supported amply by line drawings and photographs that depict anatomic or technical principles. The editors have made every attempt to minimize duplicative or repetitive discussions except when controversial or state-of-the-art issues are presented. Moreover, the editors have attempted to ensure that accurate presentations and illustrations depict properly the most complex problems confronted by the general surgeon.

Finally, in an attempt to address advances in contemporary concepts, the text has been organized to address in detail expeditious, safe, and anatomically accurate operations and incorporate standard as well as evolving surgical principles and techniques. These principles have been tested in the clinics of valid scientific knowledge and are well supported by the time-tested approaches that have been provided by practicing surgeons. The editors are excited to be able to respond to the challenge of developing a truly international text and are indeed hopeful that our readers will find this focused monograph on surgery of the esophagus and stomach to be a repository of insight, useful, and timely information.

Kirby I. Bland
Michael G. Sarr
Markus W. Büchler
Attila Csendes
Oliver James Garden
John Wong

# Contents

# Contributors

**John B. Ammori, MD**
Senior Resident Department of Surgery,
University of Michigan, Ann Arbor, MI, USA

**David A. Berg, MD**
Fellow, Colorectal Surgery, Department of Surgery,
Temple University Hospital, Philadelphia, PA, USA

**Luigi Bonavina, MD**
Associate Professor Department of Surgery,
University of Milan, Milan, Italy

**Italo Braghetto, MD, FRCS**
Professor Department of Surgery, Clinical Hospital,
University of Chile, Santiago, Chile

**Stacy A. Brethauer, MD**
Fellow, Advanced Laparoscopic and Bariatric Surgery,
Department of General Surgery, Cleveland Clinic,
Cleveland, OH, USA

**Ivan Cecconello, MD**
Professor and Chairman Department of Digestive Surgery,
São Paulo University School of Medicine, São Paulo, Brazil

**Silas M. Chikunguwo, MD, PhD, ASCP**
Fellow, Advanced Laparoscopic and Bariatric Surgery,
Department of Surgery, Cleveland Clinic Foundation,
Cleveland, OH, USA

**Kent-Man Chu, MBBS, MS, FRCS(Ed), FACS**
Professor of Surgery Department of Surgery,
University of Hong Kong, Queen Mary Hospital,
Hong Kong, China

**Willy Coosemans, MD, PhD**
Professor Department of Thoracic Surgery,
University Hospital, Leuven, Belgium

**Attila Csendes, MD, FACS (Hon)**
Professor of Surgery and Chairman Department of Surgery,
University Hospital, Santiago, Chile

**Georges Decker, MD**
Department of Thoracic Surgery, University Hospital,
Leuven, Belgium

**Paul De Leyn, MD, PhD**
Professor and Thoracic Surgeon Department of Thoracic
Surgery, University Hospital, Gasthuisberg Leuven,
Leuven, Belgium

**Ronald P. DeMatteo, MD**
Vice Chair Department of Surgery Head,
Division of General Surgical Oncology,
Memorial Sloan-Kettering Cancer Center,
New York, USA

**Daniel T. Dempsey, MD, FACS**
**George S. Peters MD, Louise C. Peters**
Chair in Surgery Department of Surgery, Temple University
School of Medicine, Philadelphia, USA

**John H. Donohue, MD**
Professor of Surgery, Division of Gastroenterologic
and General Surgery, Mayo Clinic Foundation, Rochester,
MN, USA

**Marcus Feith, MD**
University Lecturer Department of Surgery,
Technical University, Munich, Germany

**Joaquim Gama-Rodrigues, MD, PhD**
Associate Professor of Surgery,
Department of Gastroenterology, University of São Paulo,
São Paulo, Brazil

**S. Michael Griffin, MBBS, MD, FRCS(Eng), FRCS(Ed)**
Professor of Gastrointestinal Surgery,
Northern Oesophagogastric Unit, Royal Victoria Infirmary,
Newcastle upon Tyne, UK

**Jörg Hutter, MD**
Senior Physician, Department of Surgery,
Paracelsus Private Medical University, Salzburg, Austria

**Carlos Eduardo Jacob, MD, PhD**
Department of Gastroenterology, Digestive Surgery Unit,
University of São Paulo Medical School, São Paulo, Brazil

**Peter Kienle, MD**
Consultant Department of Surgery,
University of Heidelberg, Heidelberg, Germany

**Masaki Kitajima, MD, PhD, FACS, FRCS, ASA**
Professor Department of Surgery,
School of Medicine, Keio University, Tokyo, Japan

**Owen Korn, MD, FACS**
Associate Professor Department of Surgery,
Clinical Hospital University of Chile, Santiago, Chile

**Cheong J. Lee, MD**
Department of General Surgery,
University of Michigan, Ann Arbor, MI, USA

**Toni Lerut, MD, PhD**
Professor Department of Thoracic Surgery,
University Hospital, Gasthuisberg Leuven, Leuven, Belgium

**Michael W. Mulholland, MD, PhD**
**Frederick A. Coller**
Distinguished Professor, Department of Surgery,
University of Michigan, Ann Arbor, MI, USA

**Philippe Nafteux, MD**
Department of Thoracic Surgery,
University Hospital Leuven, Leuven, Belgium

**Henrique Walter Pinotti, MD**
Professor Department of Surgery, Faculty of Medicine,
University of Sao Paulo, São Paulo, Brazil

**Francesco P. Prete, MD**
Department of Surgical Sciences,
University of Foggia, Foggia, Italy

**Igor Proscurshim, BS**
Department of Gastroenterology, University of São Paulo
Medical School, São Paulo, Brazil

**Yoshiro Saikawa, MD, PhD**
Department of Surgery, School of Medicine,
Keio University, Tokyo, Japan

**Anja Schaible, MSc**
Department of Surgery,
University Hospital, Heidelberg, Germany

**Philip R. Schauer, MD**
Professor Department of General Surgery,
Cleveland Clinic, Cleveland, OH, USA

**Jonathan Shenfine, MBBS, FRCS**
Northern Oesophagogastric Unit,
Royal Victoria Infirmary, Newcastle upon Tyne, UK

**J. Rüdiger Siewert, MD**
Chairman of the Board of Directors,
University Hospital, Heidelberg, Germany

**Diane M. Simeone, MD**
Professor Department of Surgery,
University of Michigan, Ann Arbor, MI, USA

**Hubert J. Stein, MD, FACS**
Chairman Department of Surgery,
University Hospital, Salzburg, Austria

**Dirk VanRaemdonck, MD, PhD, FETCS**
Associate Professor of Surgery,
Department of Thoracic Surgery,
University Hospital, Gasthuisberg Leuven,
Leuven, Belgium

**Flavio Roberto Takeda, MD**
Research Fellow, Digestive Surgery Department,
São Paulo University School of Medicine, São Paulo, Brazil

# Part I
# Esophagus and Paraesophageal Region: Benign

# 1
# Gastroesophageal Reflux Disease

**Owen Korn**

## Pearls and Pitfalls

- Do not start treatment without a prior endoscopy to assess the esophagus and to exclude pathology of the stomach or duodenum.
- To search for intestinal metaplasia, take biopsies below the squamous-columnar line.
- An anti-reflux operation should not be offered without a complete evaluation, including endoscopy and biopsy, esophageal contrast radiology, esophageal manometry, and 24 h intraesophageal pH monitoring.
- Patients with uncomplicated gastroesophageal reflux disease (GERD) should be followed on a clinical and endoscopic basis yearly or every 2 years.
- Very symptomatic patients who do not respond to medical treatment should be evaluated thoroughly before operation is undertaken.
- Extraesophageal symptoms (asthma, cough, etc.) may be indications for anti-reflux surgery but require a detailed evaluation.
- Hiatal hernia is not synonymous with GERD.

K.I. Bland et al. (eds.), *Surgery of the Esophagus and Stomach*, DOI: 10.1007/978-1-84996-438-8_1,
© Springer Verlag London Limited 2011

- GERD with dysphagia should be assessed very carefully preoperatively, and the patient should be warned that this symptom may not improve or may even worsen.
- Do not confuse achalasia with GERD, or GERD with achalasia.

# Basic Concepts

## *Lower Esophageal Sphincter*

Clinical and manometric studies show a clear sphincteric mechanism at the gastroesophageal junction (GEJ) which constitutes a major barrier against esophageal reflux of gastric content. Despite this, the existence of an anatomic sphincter at this level has been debated for centuries. The main problem until recent years has been to demonstrate a distinct ring of a thickened circular muscle separated from the adjoining muscles by a septum of connective tissue. Such a structure does not exist at GEJ, and many studies support the concept of a 'functional' lower esophageal sphincter (LES).

Anatomic studies have demonstrated a particular orientation of the fibers of the internal muscular sheath at the GEJ forming a layer of semicircular fibers or "clasps" oriented transversally. At the GEJ, these "clasp" fibers are inserted firmly into the submucous connective tissue at the margin of contact with the oblique fibers on the opposite side. The oblique fibers replace progressively the short transverse muscle bundles of the esophagus at the greater curvature, and they build a type of muscular sling structure that covers the end of the esophagus and the anterior and posterior wall of the stomach, the so-called gastric sling fibers. Therefore, the LES is not an annular sphincter but rather formed by two muscle bundles which act in a complementary way: the "clasp" and the "oblique" muscular fibers (Fig. 1.1).

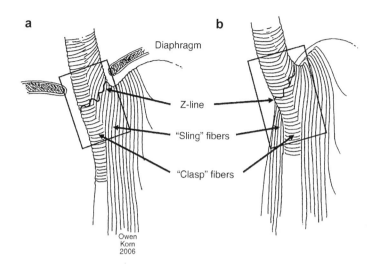

FIGURE 1.1. Schematic representation of the arrangement of the muscular fibers at the gastroesophageal junction. The area within the frame is the high pressure zone or, in other words, the lower esophageal sphincter. (**a**) lateral view; (**b**) oblique view from the lesser curve.

## Pathophysiology

Gastroesophageal reflux is linked generally to changes in dietary habits, aerophagy, and smoking is associated with many factors, such as motor disturbances of the esophagus, hiatal hernia, short esophagus, acid and/or bile reflux, delayed emptying of the stomach, and obesity, among others. Many of these factors, however, do not cause the reflux but rather are related more closely to the consequences of the reflux. From a mechanical point of view, gastroesophageal reflux in health and disease is related to loss of the barrier that confines the gastric contents to the stomach, either from inappropriate relaxation or incompetence of the LES. Transitory relaxation of the LES not mediated by swallowing, a physiologic phenomenon that allows for the release of gas from the stomach, has been cited as a factor in the majority of normal reflux events, as well as in certain pathologic situations; however, based on manometric evaluation, there is strong evidence supporting a severe mechanical compromise of the LES in patients with GERD.

*Mechanical dysfunction of the LES*: Mittal has suggested that the initial event in GERD is related most likely to frequent relaxation of the LES with reflux of gastric acid. The presence of acid in the esophagus causes esophagitis, which reduces the sphincter pressure and impairs esophageal contractility. Development of a hiatal hernia enlarges the esophageal hiatus, further impairing the sphincteric function of the crural diaphragm.

In contrast, DeMeester and his group have proposed that GERD may start in the stomach, secondary to gastric distension and delayed gastric emptying. The gastric distension causes unfolding of the LES with exposure of the terminal squamous epithelium within the LES to acid gastric juice. The length of the LES becomes no longer adequate for competency, causing a precipitous decrease in sphincter pressure, loss of the sphincter resistance, and reflux. Repetitive swallowing to clear the refluxed acid causes further gastric distention and initiates a vicious cycle.

A third potential mechanism postulated by Korn et al. involves progressive dilation of the gastroesophageal junction or cardia, probably secondary to esophagitis, which causes an irreversible change in the arrangement of the muscular bands that shape the LES, compromising LES function.

Based on these considerations, the goal of operative therapy is to restore normal competence of the intrinsic sphincter or to create a new, functional sphincter mechanism.

## Clinical Presentation

Gastroesophageal reflux is a normal physiologic event occurring generally in the post prandial period. These episodes are short-lasting, the quantity refluxed is usually small, and the refluxate is removed rapidly from the distal esophagus by esophageal clearing without damage to the esophagus. These events go unnoticed by the subject. In contrast, heartburn is the sensation caused usually by the presence of acid in the distal esophagus, while regurgitation is the clinical sensation of ascent of the refluxed material toward the mouth. These are the main two symptoms of gastroesophageal reflux, but their presence does not necessarily mean an incompetent LES, just as the absence of these symptoms does not exclude pathologic gastroesophageal reflux. Occasional heartburn is a common symptom in one of three normal subjects, while in one of ten subjects, heartburn is a common complaint.

In an attempt to establish the diagnosis of gastroesophageal disorder, we have adopted the following definition: presence of chronic symptoms lasting more than 3 months and/or existence of morphologic or functional complications of the esophagus, or well-documented, reflux-induced extra-esophageal complications (asthma, chronic cough, dysphonia, globus pharyngeus, dental deterioration, otitis, and glossitis).

Besides the classic symptoms of heartburn (95%) and regurgitation (70%), some patients com-plain of dysphagia (30%) or even retrosternal pain that can mimic cardiac pathology. Up to 20% of patients complain of isolated, extra-esophageal symptoms, such as cough, shortness of breath at night, *globus pharingeous*, dental deterioration, otitis, and glossitis.

In daily practice, patients end up in the surgeon's office most commonly referred by their physicians or gastroenterologists. Rarely, patients start with the surgeon, or they become tired of having to rely on medications and/or hear about a minimally invasive approach to operative treatment. Other scenarios involve referrals from otolaryngologists for dysphonia or "posterior laryngitis" or from pulmonologists for chronic cough or nighttime asthma. Finally, the patient with dysphagia must be approached carefully, because dysphagia is an uncommon symptom of GERD unless a complication has occurred, such as a stricture or the development of adenocarcinoma in Barrett's esophagus.

# Diagnosis

The approach to diagnosis varies a bit depending on the extent of previous evaluation. If the patient is being seen for the first time, we believe an upper endoscopy is warranted before starting therapy, although we acknowledge the existence of protocols that suggest that when faced with a patient with classic symptoms of GER, therapy can be started and the response assessed later. In contrast, in patients with a long history of "treated" GERD referred for operative treatment, a thorough re-evaluation is in order to be certain that the patient does not have achalasia, another gastroduodenal disorder, or a chronic morphologic change in the esophagus - stricture, esophageal shortening, complicated hiatal hernia, or Barrett's esophagus. Therefore, repeat endoscopy by the treating surgeon or at the least with the surgeon present to observe seems prudent.

*Upper endoscopy*: Preoperative study should include upper endoscopy to assess the state of the esophagus, investigate for Barrett's, and exclude distal lesions. A contrast radiograph of esophagus, stomach, and duodenum can be useful in the preoperative evaluation in order to detect motility disorders, esophageal stricture (length and internal diameter), anatomic dilation of the gastroesophageal junction or cardia, and presence of a true hiatal hernia, although endoscopy has almost replaced the need for a contrast study.

Endoscopy will reveal patients who have esophagus without mucosal injuries (approximately 50%), others with different degrees of esophagitis (35% of patients), and finally a group of patients with Barrett's esophagus on the first endoscopy (about 15%). The procedure should include taking biopsies above the Z line to look for the existence of chronic esophagitis, supporting the diagnosis of chronic reflux. Moreover, the endoscopist should determine whether there is ascension of the Z line or irregularities or tongues of columnar metaplasia and then should take the necessary multiple biopsies below the Z line to assess the existence of intestinal metaplasia. Besides examining the entire esophagus, the stomach and duodenum should be examined carefully for other disorders, especially for gastric cancer in those geographic areas of the world where gastric cancer has a high prevalence.

*Conventional or computerized manometric study*: Manometry of the esophagus and LES does not make the diagnosis of GERD but will support the clinical diagnosis if a mechanically incompetent LES is demonstrated (resting LES pressure ≤6 mmHg, total length ≤20 mm, or LES abdominal length ≤10 mm); these findings suggest a severe anatomic and functional abnormality of the sphincter. In addition, the amplitude and coordination of esophageal contractions provide potentially useful information of esophageal function, especially if esophageal contractile activity is diminished markedly; the latter finding may alter the extent of operative fundoplication.

*24 h intraesophageal pH-probe monitoring (24 h pH study)*: This test is actually the "gold standard" to establish the presence of pathologic gastroesophageal reflux, defined as the excessive duration of exposure of the esophageal lumen to gastric juice. The study is performed by placing a small diameter pH electrode, introduced transnasally, 5 cm proximal to the LES, which has been located previously by manometry.

A special, computerized program allows analysis of the stored data and gives a profile of the number, duration, and timing of reflux episodes culminating in a score which combines six different parameters. A combined score ≤14 is normal. Probably the most useful value is the total time per 24 h during which intraesophageal pH is <4, with normal being ≤4% (55 min). In addition, it is important to correlate the relationship between reflux periods and symptoms. This test represents the most objective means to establish presence of a pathologic gastroesophageal reflux, and many surgeons believe that every candidate for an anti-reflux operation should have this test prior to operation.

*24 h bilirubin monitoring of the distal esophagus*: The importance of duodenal reflux into the esophagus in the pathophysiology of GERD and its complications is also well recognized. Although this test is not a routine procedure for most patients with GERD, it should be considered in patients with suspicion of duodenal reflux, especially in patients with Barrett's esophagus or in patients with symptoms of gastroesophageal reflux but with a normal 24 h pH study.

*Impedance study*: Recently, impedance technology with the capability of detecting all types of reflux (acid, non-acid, liquid, mixed, and air) has been developed. Recent work has shown that nonacid reflux can be an important clinical problem with over half of the reflux events not detected by pH studies. The additional information provided by impedance technology is likely to have a major impact on our understanding and clinical management of patients with GERD. While experience to date is limited, this technology may prove to be the best assessment of sphincter competency.

# Medical Treatment and Operative Indications in GERD

Today, practically all patients with GERD can be managed symptomatically with medical treatment by modifying lifestyle and dietary habits, plus the use of proton pump inhibitors with or without prokinetics. Medical therapy, however, is mainly symptomatic, designed to inhibit acid production, minimize heartburn, and improve esophagitis, but it does not stop the reflux, because it is not able to restore sphincter function. In contrast, reflux of duodenal content is not controlled, and regurgitation of gastric contents during exercise or when recumbent can be very bothersome and persists in spite of complete acid blockade. As medical therapy accomplishes symptomatic well-being in most all patients, it becomes very difficult to accept failure of medical treatment as an indication for operation. Indeed, when the indication for operative intervention is a failure of medical management, the patient requires very careful and comprehensive review.

The ideal candidate for an anti-reflux operation is a patient with typical symptoms of heartburn and/or regurgitation, with pH-proven, pathologic esophageal acid exposure and who is dependent on proton-pump inhibitors for symptomatic relief. A multivariate analysis of the factors predicting a successful outcome after laparoscopic Nissen fundoplication identified these three parameters as the most important preoperative predictive factors: the 24 h pH probe study, typical symptoms of gastroesophageal reflux, and a good response to medical treatment (Table 1.1). Considering the previous statement, we believe that current indications in GERD for an anti-reflux operation are:

1.  Recurrent symptomatology appearing early after stopping appropriate medical treatment
2.  Dependence or increasing requirements of acid-suppressive drugs
3.  Persistent and/or progressive GERD despite active medical treatment
4.  Young patients obliged to medical treatment for life
5.  A mechanically incompetent LES
6.  Laryngo-respiratory symptoms secondary to GERD
7.  Alterations in esophageal motility
8.  True hiatal hernia and GERD
9.  Severe abnormal acid reflux on 24 h pH probe study

TABLE 1.1. Predictor of outcome after laparoscopic fundoplication: stepwise logistic regression results in 199 patients* (Adapted from Campos et al., 1999. With permission of Springer Science + Business Media).

| Predictor | Adjusted odds ratio* (95% confidence intervals) | Wald's P-value |
|---|---|---|
| 24 h pH composite score | 5.4 (1.9–15.3) | <0.001 |
| Typical primary symptoms | 5.1 (1.9–13.7) | <0.001 |
| Good response to medical therapy | 3.3 (1.3–8.7) | <0.03 |

*Odds ratios and corresponding P values are adjusted for all other factors in the model.

For all these indications, probably the most difficult indication to define clearly is persistent and/or progressive disease. These patients usually are well-managed with medical therapy; nevertheless, clinical experience suggests that they often end up at the surgeon's door. Characteristically, these patients become dependent on drugs and experience cycles of remission and relapse. The most important issue is to recognize some of the risk factors that seem to define a more severe clinical profile, such as:

1. Severe mechanical defect of the LES established by manometric study
2. Severe erosive esophagitis at endoscopy
3. Supine reflux
4. Mixed reflux
5. Persistent esophageal stricture
6. Barrett's esophagus, especially with any element of dysplasia

In early stages of GERD, it may be very difficult to demonstrate a mechanically incompetent LES according to standard manometric parameters. As the disease progresses and lesions and/or complications become evident, the finding of a mechanically defective sphincter is common, being present in more than 90% of patients with Barrett's esophagus. Although it is argued that damage to the sphincter is either primary or secondary to the esophageal damage, what is clear is that sphincter damage cannot be recovered and is irreversible despite aggressive medical therapy. Anti-reflux surgery can, however, restore or improve lost sphincter function when there is still a remnant of an intrinsic sphincter. In these cases, anti-reflux surgery offers a therapeutic alternative that is more efficient than any medical therapy and eventually may change the natural course of the disease.

## Operative Treatment of GERD

The goals of operative intervention and the techniques used to reach that goal are detailed as follows:

- Fundoplication (Nissen) or cardial calibration (Hill-Larraín)
  - Restores or recovers the function of a mechanically incompetent LES and narrows or calibrates the dilated gastroesophageal junction
  - Increases resting LES pressure, decreasing the frequency of reflux
  - Optimizes sphincteric competence
- Posterior Gastropexy
  - Fixes the abdominal esophagus below the diaphragmatic hiatus
  - Maintains the distal esophagus subject to intraabdominal pressure
  - Prevents para-esophagic hiatal hernia
- Closure of the diaphragm pillars
  - Increases resistance to reflux during increases in abdominal pressure
  - Complement sphincteric action
  - Avoids paraesophageal hiatal hernia

According to the majority of experts in anti-reflux surgery, there are no differences in the operative treatment of a patient with acid gastroesophageal reflux with or without esophagitis from that of a patient with Barrett's esophagus. Most anti-reflux procedures employ some type of fundoplication technique, usually the Nissen fundoplication, with satisfactory results. In contrast, we believe that the operative treatment of the patient with acid GERD should differ from that of a patient with long-segment or complicated Barrett's esophagus, because clinically and pathophysiologically they represent different disease processes. The patient with acid GERD usually has a sphincter less damaged mechanically, a not very dilated gastroesophageal junction and diaphragmatic hiatus, a more or less preserved esophageal motility, and a pathologic predominance of acid reflux. In contrast, Barrett's esophagus usually occurs at a later state of chronic gastroesophageal reflux, and many (including the author) believe that reflux of bile should be a major target of the anti-reflux procedure.

In addition, a number of procedures have been developed to treat the "shortened" esophagus, often by a Collis-Nissen technique performed laparoscopically. In our experience, we have never observed the so-called short esophagus of a magnitude described in the literature and never more than 2 cm. Based on our experience, after complete dissection of the esophagogastric junction, we have always found the gastroesophageal sphincter to be in an intraabdominal location. Also, in the case of true hiatal hernias, with the hernia sac and the part of the stomach proximal to the hiatus, it has always been possible to relocate the LES within the abdomen.

## Outcome

To be successful, anti-reflux surgery must provide long-term relief of reflux symptoms and not create complications or complaints secondary to the operation. Operative or postoperative complications (splenic injury, hemorrhage, pulmonary complications, temporary dysphagia) occur on average in 8–10% of patients, and the rate of conversion to an open procedure is about 2% in accomplished hands (range 1–10%) Mortality is uncommon, but patients should be warned that they will have some dysphagia for 1–2 months postoperatively. With the use of fundoplicature techniques in patients with non-complicated acid GERD, the results in our group in the long term (5 or 10 years) show 85% good to excellent results, comparable to the data of most authors in the literature. Objective studies have shown that >90% of patients will have negative pH studies 1–3 years after laparoscopic Nissen fundoplication (Table 1.2). It is important to point out that all series of anti-reflux techniques should be assessed in the long range, because in 2–3 years most of the patients with simple reflux are clinically well.

Finally, we should point out that GERD, given its frequency and importance especially with today's possibilities of study and therapy, is at the center of interest of many groups. For that same reason, it has been exposed to the interplay of

TABLE 1.2. 24 h pH studies after laparoscopic Nissen fundoplication (Reprinted from Peters et al., 2000).

| Primary author | pH-negative patients | Follow-up (months) |
| --- | --- | --- |
| Hinder | 21/24 (87%) | 3–12 |
| Hunter | 49/54 (91%) | 12 |
| Watson | 42/48 (87%) | 3 |
| Peters | 26/28 (93%) | 21 |
| Csendes | 35/45 (77) | 40 |

diverse interests in different medical and surgical fields as well as in the technologic industries. Thus, those treating these patients need to be extremely cautious and critical of all new therapies (operative, endoscopic, etc.) and to maintain a critical attitude based on objective and controlled studies and not based only on impressions.

## Selected Readings

Campos GM, Peters JH, DeMeester TR et al. (1999) Multi-variate analysis of factors predicting outcome after laparoscopic Nissen fundoplication. J Gastrointest Surg 3:292–300

Darling G, Deschamps C (2005) Technical controversies in fundoplication surgery. Thorac Surg Clin 15:437–444

Dent J, Holloway RH, Toouli J, Dodds WJ (1988) Mechanisms of lower oesophageal sphincter incompetence in patients with symptomatic gastroesophageal reflux. Gut 29:1020–1028

Kahrilas PJ, Lee TJ (2005) Pathophysiology of gastroesophageal reflux disease. Thorac Surg Clin 15:323–333

Korn O, Stein HJ, Richter T, Liebermann-Meffert D (1997) Gastroesophageal sphincter: a model. Dis Esoph 10:105–109

Peters JH, Hagen JA, DeMeester SR et al. (2000) Advances in surgical techniques and technology: a decade of laparoscopic Nissen fundoplication. Contemp Surg 56:138–151

Skinner DB (1985) Pathophysiology of gastroesophageal reflux. Ann Surg 202:546–556

Watson TJ, Peters JH (2005) Evaluation of esophageal function for anti-reflux surgery. Gastrointest Endosc Clin N Am 15:347–360

# 2
# Paraesophageal Hiatus Hernia

**Luigi Bonavina**

## Pearls and Pitfalls

- Paraesophageal (type II) hiatus hernia represents a distinct anatomic and clinic entity requiring a unique therapeutic strategy, and is differentiated from the more common type I (sliding) hiatus hernia.
- All symptomatic patients, in the absence of prohibitive operative risk, should undergo elective repair to prevent life-threatening complications, such as obstruction, strangulation, perforation, and bleeding.
- Extended transmediastinal dissection and complete sac excision are mandatory to reduce the stomach and the distal esophagus safely into the abdomen; a Collis gastroplasty is necessary only infrequently.
- The anterior sac can be left attached to the cardia and used for downward traction; identify and avoid injury to the anterior vagus nerve.
- A retrogastric lipoma is constant and should be excised to enable complete dissection of the diaphragmatic pillars behind the esophagus; identify and avoid injury to the posterior vagus nerve.
- Crural repair with prosthetic patch onlay has the potential to reduce the recurrence rate but insufficient data are available at present to confirm safety, best prosthetic, and long-term effectiveness.

K.I. Bland et al. (eds.), *Surgery of the Esophagus and Stomach*, DOI: 10.1007/978-1-84996-438-8_2, © Springer-Verlag London Limited 2011

- The addition of a Nissen-or Toupet-fundoplication techniques reduces the incidence of postoperative gastroesophageal reflux.
- The role of a concomitant anterior gastropexy constructed to prevent intraabdominal gastric volvulus and recurrent hernia remains controversial.
- Laparoscopic repair is feasible and remains the approach of choice in patients with paraesophageal hiatus hernia.

Hiatal hernias are heterogeneous anatomic and clinical entities. Classification into four types is widely accepted. Sliding hernia is the result of an upward migration of the esophagogastric junction into the mediastinum (type I hiatus hernia). Paraesophageal hiatus hernia (type II hiatus hernia) occurs as a result of an anterior defect in the diaphragmatic hiatus leading to an upward dislocation of the gastric fundus alongside the cardia. Subsequent progressive enlargement of the hiatus and the hernia sac leads to a mixed paraesophageal and sliding hernia (type III hiatus hernia) which may evolve to the final stage characterized by a complete, intrathoracic, "upside-down" stomach. Therefore, the distinction between type II and type III hernias is somewhat artificial because they are considered a continuous disease spectrum. Infrequently, the colon can migrate into the hernia sac (type IV hiatus hernia).

Approximately 10% of hiatus hernias have a paraesophageal component, and among these patients, 90% have a mixed type III hernia.

The true incidence of paraesophageal hernia in the overall population is unknown because of minimal or even absence of symptoms in many individuals. The majority of patients with paraesophageal hernia are elderly females who often present with multiple comorbidities.

A progressive, structural deterioration of the phrenoesophageal ligament may explain the higher incidence of paraesophageal hernia in the older age group. Anatomic changes involve thinning of the upper fascial layer of the ligament (continuation of the endothoracic fascia) and loss of elasticity of the lower fascial layer (continuation of the transversalis fascia). In a mixed type III hernia, because of continuous stretching in the cranial direction from intra-abdominal pressure, the esophagogastric junction migrates into the mediastinum through the widened hiatus; a portion of the lesser curvature of the stomach accompanies the esophagogastric junction and forms part of the wall of the hernia sac. Consequently, the lower esophageal sphincter lies outside the abdominal cavity and is unaffected by its environmental pressures. As the size of the hernia increases, the greater curvature will roll up along the left side of the esophagogastric junction into the posterior mediastinum. The stomach can become incarcerated above the diaphragm; if a 180° rotation occurs around its longitudinal axis, this forms an organo-axial volvulus or, less commonly, if the rotation occurs around the transverse axis, it is called a mesoaxial volvulus (Fig. 2.1a, b). These volvuli can cause a number of mechanical complications resulting in vascular congestion of the gastric mucosa, gastric outlet obstruction, and impairment of pulmonary function due to displacement of the lung (Table 2.1).

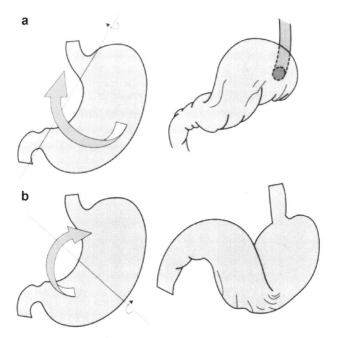

FIGURE 2.1. Schematic view of the organo-axial (**a**) and of the meso-axial gastric volvulus (**b**).

TABLE 2.1. Classification and characteristics of hiatal hernias.

| Hernia type | Location of EGJ | Hernia contents | Size | Rotation | Spontaneous reducibility | Major complications |
|---|---|---|---|---|---|---|
| I (sliding) | Intrathoracic | Fundus | 1–5 cm | None | Commonly complete | Reflux esophagitis, Barrett's esophagus |
| II (true paraesophageal) | Intraabdominal | Fundus | 1–5 cm | None or organoaxial | Often fixed | Obstruction, strangulation, perforation, bleeding |
| III (mixed) | Intrathoracic | Fundus + body | >50% of stomach | Organoaxial and mesoaxial | Fixed | Obstruction, strangulation, perforation, bleeding |
| IV (mixed + other contents) | Intrathoracic | Fundus + body + other | >50% of stomach + colon | Organoaxial and mesoaxial | Fixed | Obstruction, strangulation, perforation, bleeding |

# Clinical Presentation

Up to 50% of patients with paraesophageal hiatus hernia are asymptomatic or complain of only minor symptoms. Typical chronic symptoms include postprandial distress (epigastric fullness, nausea, intermittent vomiting, chest discomfort, dyspnea), heartburn, regurgitation, dysphagia, and hematemesis. Acute symptoms can mimic an acute myocardial infarction and develop as a consequence of complete gastric outflow obstruction. Anemia secondary to chronic bleeding and lung dysfunction secondary to aspiration are the most typical signs associated with paraesophageal hiatus hernia (Table 2.2). In as many as 20% of patients, the clinical presentation of a massive and incarcerated paraesophageal hernia may be urgent or emergent. Acute distress with chest pain and inability to vomit can occur as a result of complete obstruction, strangulation, or perforation of the intrathoracic stomach.

TABLE 2.2. Symptoms associated with paraesophageal hiatus hernia in 141 patients (Data from Hiebert, 1995).

| Symptoms | % |
|---|---|
| Epigastric fullness | 83 |
| Post-prandial pain | 75 |
| Regurgitation | 60 |
| Heartburn | 57 |
| Nausea/vomiting | 41 |
| Aspiration | 41 |
| Dysphagia | 38 |
| Bleeding | 32 |
| Respiratory embarrassment | 25 |
| Complete obstruction | 13 |

## *Diagnosis*

A paraesophageal hiatus hernia is often suspected on the basis of an abnormality on an incidental chest x-ray because of a retrocardiac air bubble with or without an air-fluid level on the lateral view (Fig. 2.2). A barium swallow confirms the diagnosis (Fig. 2.3a, b). Computed tomography (CT) of the chest and abdomen are of little value in the diagnosis, but may provide information on surrounding anatomy and will exclude concomitant pathology (Fig. 2.4). Upper gastrointestinal endoscopy is mandatory in all patients to exclude the presence of esophagitis, Barrett's esophagus, or associated adenocarcinoma. A mixed type III hernia can be identified on retroversion of the endoscope by noting a gastric

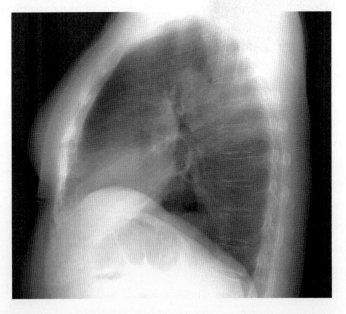

FIGURE 2.2. Lateral chest film: retrocardiac air-fluid level is suggestive of paraesophageal hernia.

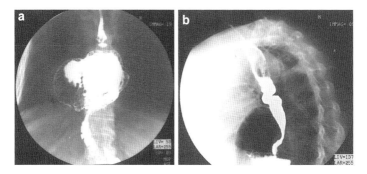

FIGURE 2.3. (**a, b**) Barium swallow study showing a mixed type III paraesophageal hiatus hernia.

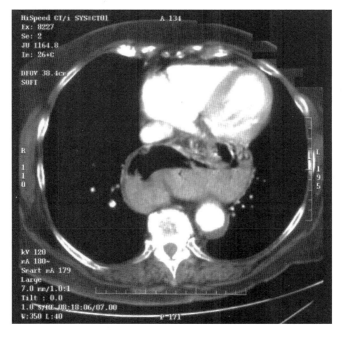

FIGURE 2.4. Chest CT showing almost complete dislocation of the stomach in the lower mediastinal compartment.

pouch lined with rugal folds above the diaphragm, and the gastroesophageal junction entering about midway up the side of the pouch (Fig. 2.5). In some circumstances, due to the organoaxial rotation of the stomach, it can be difficult to advance the endoscope into the antropyloric region. Preoperative esophageal function studies are typically unnecessary when symptoms are related clearly to gastric outlet obstruction and distension of the intrathoracic stomach. However, if dysphagia is an accompanying symptom, an esophageal manometry should be performed to rule out achalasia. Because many of these patients are elderly, noninvasive cardiac stress testing should also be considered before planning an operation.

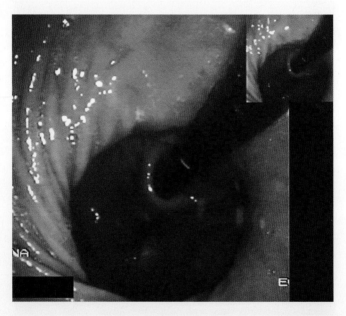

FIGURE 2.5. Typical appearance of a type III paraesophageal hiatus hernia on endoscopic retroversion: a gastric pouch lined with rugal folds is seen to extend above the crura impression; the gastroesophageal junction enters about midway up the side of the pouch.

# Treatment

Operative repair is currently the only effective therapy for paraesophageal hiatus hernia. It has long been advised that any medically fit patient should undergo operative correction irrespective of symptoms or age. This recommendation was based on reports suggesting a 30% risk of developing life-threatening complications with these types of hernia, and an associated increased risk of mortality with emergent intervention. Some authors, however, advocate a careful watchful waiting strategy in selected asymptomatic or minimally symptomatic patients based on the apparent reduced morbidity and mortality of urgent/emergent intervention compared with previous estimates.

Traditional repair of paraesophageal hiatus hernia has consisted of left thoracotomy or laparotomy. The minimally invasive laparoscopic approach has gained wide acceptance quickly over the past decade. The main advantages of a laparoscopic approach for patients include less postoperative discomfort, earlier mobilization, reduced perioperative morbidity, and shorter hospital stay and convalescence. It is imperative that the laparoscopic repair follow the same surgical principles adopted in the traditional operation, i.e., complete tension-free reduction of the stomach and distal esophagus in the abdominal cavity en bloc with the hernia sac, and the appropriate repair of the crura. Even in the laparoscopic era, however, several areas of controversy persist in the management of paraesophageal hiatus hernia. These include the treatment of a short esophagus, the importance of sac excision, the role of a prosthesis in the repair of the crura defect, the need for a fundoplication, and the need for an anterior gastropexy.

# Technique of Laparoscopic Repair

The patient is placed in the dorsal lithotomy position using reverse Trendelenburg (20–30) as needed. The surgeon is positioned between the patient's legs. The pneumoperitoneum is induced by means of a Veress needle placed in the umbilicus or in the left hypochondrium in obese patients and maintained at an average of 13 mmHg; it is wise to lower insufflation pressures to 9 mmHg occasionally to avoid hypercarbia and hypotension in an elderly, frail patient. Five trocars, two 10 mm and three 5 mm ones, are used for the operation. The first 10 mm port is placed in the midline about 15 cm below the xiphoid process and is used for the 30° scope. The second 10 mm port is placed under direct vision higher in the left midclavicular line and is used for the needle-holder, the ultrasonic shears, and the irrigation-aspiration device. A 5 mm port is placed at the same level in the right midclavicular line for the operating grasper. Two additional 5 mm trocars are placed just below the xiphoid process for the liver retractor and in the left midclavicular line at the level of umbilicus for the stomach retractor. A common mistake is to place the ports too low in the abdominal wall, thereby making the mediastinal dissection more difficult. The operation starts by gently pulling the gastric fundus in the caudal direction with atraumatic graspers and dissecting the peritoneum off the free edge of the left crura as far posteriorly as possible. Inserting a rolled-up piece of gauze at the level of the gastrosplenic ligament provides additional retraction and improves visualization of this area. Blunt and sharp dissection is used to tease gently the entire hernia sac out of the mediastinum by entering the avascular plane between the endoabdominal fascia and the muscle body of the left crus. Accurate hemostasis is achieved with the ultrasonic shears. Both the surgeon and the anesthesiologist should be aware of the risk of pneumothorax at this time. The dissection continues anteriorly toward the right crus. The redundant hernia sac is left attached to the anterior aspect of the esophagogastric junction, purposely, because this strong tissue can then be used for effective gastric retraction. The lesser omentum is then opened and the right crus identified. The dissection continues posteriorly where a large lipoma is usually identified and needs to be resected to allow creation of a window behind the esophagus. Working through this window from the right side may help not only to recognize and preserve the posterior vagal nerve, but also to complete the dissection of the left crus and the posterior aspect of the gastric fundus. At this point, the distal esophagus can be encircled with a soft drain. The mediastinal cavity is inspected for hemostasis, and further blunt/sharp dissection is performed to ensure that an adequate length of the esophagus has been reduced into the abdomen without any tension. On rare occasions, a Collis gastroplasty may be necessary. The standard posterior crural repair is performed using 4–6 interrupted sutures of 2-0 polypropylene using extracorporeal knots. Teflon pledgets can be used to buttress these sutures. A synthetic prosthesis can be used to reinforce the crural repair. In selected patients we have used a onlay composite mesh, such as the Crurasoft patch (Bard) and the Parietex composite (Sofradim), fixed to the crura with a few stitches. Others have used a bioprosthesis. A fundoplication is added routinely in these patients regardless of the presence of reflux before the operation. In elderly patients, we prefer to perform a Toupet fundoplication which encompasses the posterior 180–270° of the distal esophagus. The first two stitches fix the apex of the gastric fundus to the left and the right crura, respectively; four more sutures are then placed between the gastric wall and each side of the esophagus. An anterior gastropexy can be added to the repair when the reduced stomach is prone to recurrent torsion. A closed-suction drain is placed in the mediastinum, and another drain under the left liver. All patients undergo an oral soluble contrast study on postoperative day 1, and a clear liquid diet is started. Most patients are discharged on postoperative day 2 or 3.

## Outcome

Laparoscopic approach for paraesophageal hiatus hernia is feasible, safe, and effective. Postoperative complications are similar to those seen after conventional antireflux surgery, except for a higher reported incidence of esophageal and gastric injuries. Durability of the repair is still the critical issue.

Most series have used primarily symptomatic follow-up and have reported recurrence rates of 0–5%. However, postoperative radiographic studies have found high rates of asymptomatic anatomic recurrence, ranging from 23% to 46%. Dissection of the hernia sac promotes safe mobilization of the esophagus and may improve the short and long-term success rate. It is not clear whether the use of a prosthesis to reinforce the crural repair outweighs the potential risk of visceral erosion, particularly with a synthetic polypropylene mesh. In conclusion, laparoscopic repair remains the approach of choice in patients with paraesophageal hiatus hernia. There is an ongoing need to assess mechanisms of late recurrence and reduce its incidence.

## Selected Readings

DeMeester T, Bonavina L (1989) Paraesophageal hiatal hernia. In: Nyhus L, Condon R (eds) Hernia. Lippincott, Philadelphia, pp 684–693

Ferri L, Feldman L, Stanbridge D et al. (2005) Should laparoscopic paraesophageal hernia repair be abandoned in favor of the open approach? Surg Endosc 19:4–8

Hashemi M, Peters J, DeMeester T et al. (2000) Laparoscopic repair of large type III hiatal hernia: objective follow-up reveals high recurrence rate. J Am Coll Surg 190:539–547

Hiebert C (1995) Massive incarcerated hiatal hernia. In: Pearson FG et al. (eds) Esophageal surgery. Churchill Livingstone, New York, pp 267–271

Skinner D, Belsey R (1988): Types II, IIA, III, and para-esophageal hiatal heria. In: Management of esophageal disease, Saunders, Philadelphia, pp 631–639

Stylopoulos N, Gazelle G, Rattner D (2002) Paraesophageal hernias: operation or observation? Ann Surg 236: 492–500

Watson D, Davies N, Devitt P, Jamieson G (1999) Importance of dissection of the hernial sac in laparoscopic surgery for large hiatal hernias. Arch Surg 134:1069–1073

Wo J, Branum J, Hunter J et al. (1996) Clinical features of type III (mixed) paraesophageal hernia. Am J Gastroenterol 91:914–916

# 3
# Barrett's Esophagus

**Attila Csendes**

## Pearls and Pitfalls

- Suspect Barrett's esophagus (BE) in a white, adult, middle-aged patient with a long-standing history of gastroesophageal reflux.
- BE is a frequent histologic finding in the distal esophagus, provided routine biopsy samples are taken.
- BE is a preneoplastic disease with an annual incidence of adenocarcinoma is 0.5–0.8%.
- Adenocarcinoma can appear in patients with short-segment BE.
- Short-segment BE is four times more frequent than long-segment BE.
- Adenocarcinoma of the distal esophagus originating from BE has increased 500% in the last three decades.
- The end-point of medical treatment is the control of symptoms, which is not equivalent to control of acid and duodenal reflux into the distal esophagus.
- Increased experimental evidence shows that the mixture of acid and duodenal juice refluxing into the esophagus is deleterious and carcinogenic.
- Low-grade dysplasia is a good index for eventual development of high grade dysplasia or adenocarcinoma.
- Antireflux surgery seems to be superior to medical treatment but does not prevent the appearance of adenocarcinoma.

K.I. Bland et al. (eds.), *Surgery of the Esophagus and Stomach*, DOI: 10.1007/978 1 84996 438 8_3,
© Springer-Verlag London Limited 2011

- Nearly 50% of patients with high-grade dysplasia may already have an early localized or multifocal adenocarcinoma.
- In patients with high grade dysplasia, endoscopic ablation is a good alternative to esophagectomy, although residual BE and even adenocarcinoma may develop beneath the new squamous epithelium.
- Nissen fundoplication is an excellent operation for patients with short-segment BE, with regression of intestinal metaplasia in about 50% of patients.
- In patients with long-segment BE, acid suppression and duodenal diversion seems a more appropriate alternative to Nissen fundoplication, producing permanent control of acid and duodenal reflux and a change in the natural history of BE, by eliminating the appearance of adenocarcinoma.

Barrett's esophagus (BE) is an acquired condition in which the distal squamous epithelium of the esophagus is replaced by a columnar mucosa containing intestinal metaplasia due to chronic gastroesophageal reflux disease (GERD). In 1950, Barrett described the presence of a peptic ulcer with a distal tubular segment of intrathoracic stomach, with the presence of a congenitally short esophagus. Others, however, found in this "intrathoracic tubular stomach" the presence of mucosal glands in the submucosa, more typical of the esophagus and not of an intrathoracic stomach, clarifying this as columnar lined epithelium of the esophagus and showed it to be associated with hiatal hernia. Classically, a diagnosis of BE required that at least 3 cm of the distal esophagus be lined by metaplastic columnar epithelium, which is now called long-segment BE. By contrast, the existence of "short segment" BE, involving columnar mucosa plus intestinal metaplasia of either circumferential increase (>1cm) or one or more tongues (>1cm) or a combination of these findings, but always less than 3cm in length, is recognized increasingly and is four times more common than "long-segment" BE. The main importance of BE is that it predisposes the development of adenocarcinoma.

# Epidemiology

BE is found in 1–2% of unselected normal population under-going endoscopy and in 6–20% of patients submitted to endo-scopic evaluation for symptoms of GERD. Intestinal metaplasia of the cardia, which is the histologic finding of intestinal meta-plasia in otherwise normal endoscopy (and therefore not true BE) is found in 12% of patients with GERD, without the endoscopic findings of a BE. Its importance and future behav-ior have not been evaluated nor clarified (Fig. 3.1).

The incidence of BE has increased markedly since 1970, due in part to the increase in endoscopic procedures. Autopsy studies suggest that for each known case of long-segment BE,

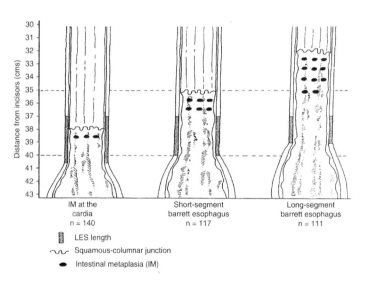

FIGURE 3.1. Schematic representation of endoscopic histologic and manometric studies in patients with cardia intestinal metaplasia (IM), short-segment Barrett's esophagus, and long-segment Barrett's esophagus. The length and location of the lower esophageal sphincter is established clearly, as well as the oral displacement of the squamo-columnar junction, with a 2 cm "shortening" of the esophagus in patients with long-segment BE.

there are 20 additional unrecognized patients. BE is more frequent among white, Anglo Saxons, Europeans, and the Hispanic population and is much less common among the African and Asian population. In the last 3 decades, there has been a 500% increase in the incidence of adenocarcinoma arising from BE with the majority located at the distal esophagus, while squamous-cell carcinoma has decreased. The reason for this increase in unknown. Epidemiologic studies have identified a variety of risk factors for the development of esophageal adenocarcinoma: the presence of BE is the only clearly recognized risk factor. Severe, long-standing symptoms of reflux, increased body mass index, and dietary and environmental issues (smoking and a diet low in fresh fruit) are also important factors. The precise incidence of adenocarcinoma in patients with BE is uncertain, varying from 1/52 to 1/297 patient-years of follow up. Recent studies suggest that the annual risk is 0.5–0.8%.

## Pathogenesis

In most patients, BE develops in the setting of chronic symptomatic GERD, in which two metaplastic events occur (Fig. 3.2). The first involves a phenotypic transformation of squamous cells to cardiac mucosa secondary to chronic acid reflux. The second metaplastic change involves the appearance of intestinal goblet cells without the normalabsorptive capacity(incompleteintestinalmetaplasia),believed secondary to duodeno-esophageal reflux and genetic predisposition. Clinical and endoscopic evidence cannot determine precisely when the condition developed or its extent. Many investigators believe that BE usually develops to its full extent all at once, and that there is no substantial progress in length with time.

BE is associated clearly with a mixture of severe acid reflux and duodenal content refluxing into the distal esophagus. In animal experiments, acid reflux alone is a rare cause of adenocarcinoma of the esophagus, while mixed reflux is associated clearly with development of adenocarcinoma. Bile

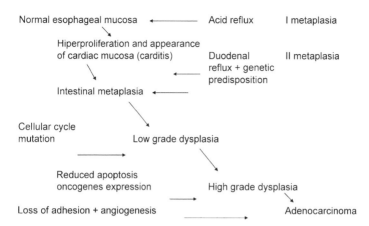

FIGURE 3.2. Development of Barrett's esophagus and adenocarcinoma through the occurrence of two metaplastic changes. The first metaplastic change is basically a phenotypic change, while the second metaplastic change is a genotypic change.

salts are probably the noxious component in the refluxed duodenal juice, being pH-dependent (Fig. 3.3). For bile salts to cause injury, they must be soluble and unionized. A pH less than 2 produces irreversible precipitation; however, at a pH of 3–5, a mixture of bile salt and bile acids is present and can rapidly cross the mucosal cell membrane and destroy the mitochondria. Other abnormalities found in patients with BE are the presence of an incompetent lower esophageal sphincter (LES) and an alteration in esophageal motility producing a disturbance in esophageal clearance.

Three types of columnar epithelia have been described in BE: (1) specialized columnar epithelium (intestinal metaplasia) with a villiform surface and intestinal-type crypts lined by mucus-secreting cells and goblet cells, (2) fundic type epithelium containing chief and parietal cells, and (3) junctional type epithelium with a foveolar surface and mucus-secreting cells. The latter two epithelial cells can be found normally at the cardia or esophagogastric junction (EG). The cell of origin of BE remains unclear, but evidence points to multipotential stem cells as the site of origin of BE. There

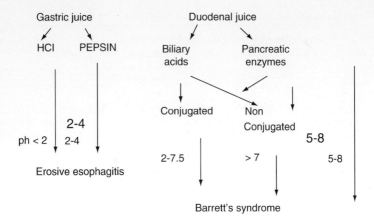

FIGURE 3.3. Harmful effect of the gastric and duodenal juice to the distal esophagus. Experimentally, gastric juice alone at pH 2 to 4, by activating pepsin, is able to produce only erosive esophagitis. Bile salts present at the gastric lumen are pH dependant and at pH 3 to 5, together with acid, are noxious to esophageal mucosa producing BE and even adenocarcinoma.

are some problems in the clear definition of Barrett's esophagus.

The precise identification of the gastroesophageal junction can be controversial. The anatomic end of the esophagus corresponds to the distal limit of the sling and clasp fibers of the lower esophageal sphincter. Radiologically, it is difficult to locate precisely. To the physiologists, the esophagogastric junction corresponds to the limit of the LES. For the endoscopists, the E-G junction corresponds to the proximal margin of the gastric folds.

The endoscopic and manometric landmarks may be imprecise due to the constant physiologic movement of the esophago-gastric junction.

In normal subjects, the squamous-columnar junction is located in the mid-portion of the LES, which means that nearly 15 mm of the final portion of the abdominal esophagus is covered by gastric or columnar mucosa. This squamo-columnar junction is displaced orally with severe reflux.

# Clinical Features

It is impossible to confirm the presence or the diagnosis of a BE by only clinical means; endoscopy and biopsy are required. BE is usually discovered in middle aged adults (mean age 55 years old) with a slight male predominance. Symptoms of GERD are present usually for at least 10 or more years; however, 11% of patients with short-segment BE and 2% with long-segment BE are truly asymptomatic and are found only by endoscopic evaluation.

Hiatal hernia, as well as complications such a peptic ulcer of the esophagus or strictures, are more common in patients with long-segment BE compared with patients with short-segment BE. The presence of dysplasia at the metaplastic mucosa is 3–4 times greater in patients with long-segment BE.

# Diagnosis

Endoscopic examination with multiple biopsies is required to establish the diagnosis of a BE. Endoscopically, Barrett's mucosa has a salmon-pink appearance almost identical to that of gastric mucosa. The columnar-lined mucosa extends proximally up the esophagus in irregular, finger-like or tongue projections or, less frequently, as a circumferential sheet. There may be isolated or heterotopic islands of gastric mucosa surrounded by squamous epithelium in the distal esophagus. The presence of goblet cells in cardiac mucosa stained with Alcien blue at pH 2.5 confirms the existence of a Barrett's mucosa. Intestinal metaplasia is found in only 1/3 of the patients with "short-segment" BE. The prevalence of intestinal metaplasia increases in parallel with the length of the columnar epithelium, and when BE is >6 cm, practically 100% of patients have intestinal metaplasia. Thus, BE is often suspected at the time of endoscopy but not always confirmed.

What does this mean? At the time of endoscopy, landmarks should be evaluated and defined carefully. If the squamo-columnar junction is 10 mm or more above the level of the esophagogastric junction defined as the proximal margin of gastric folds under partial insufflations, biopsy specimens should be obtained, and if goblet cells are present, the patient is considered to have BE and should be placed under medical treatment and surveillance. The risk of adenocarcinoma is increased to 1/50 to 1/250 patient-years of follow up, which means a risk 30-to 120-fold greater than the general population. The annual incidence of adenocarcinoma varies between 0.5–1% among patients with BE. Other laboratory investigations should be considered in patients with BE, especially in those who are candidates for surgical therapy. The prevalence of a mechanically defective sphincter on manometry is greater in patients with BE and parallels the length of the columnar mucosa. Similarly, poor esophageal contractility also is present often, and clearance of the esophagus may be delayed. Acid reflux and duodenal reflux are also greater in patients with long-segment BE compared with patients with short-segment BE. Therefore, not only acid but bile and pancreatic juice may be present in the refluxed material.

## Medical Treatment

The main goal of medical therapy is to maintain patients with BE free of symptoms and to heal esophagitis. Proton pump inhibitors result consistently in relief of symptoms and healing of esophagitis. But symptom control is not necessarily equivalent to normalization of acid or duodenal exposure of the distal esophagus, despite use of high-dose proton pump inhibitors; 15–40% of patients still have pathologic acid reflux while receiving 20 mg of Omeprazole twice daily. The same phenomenon occurs with duodeno-esophageal reflux, which is not controlled at all by proton pump inhibitors. Nevertheless, aggressive and effective acid suppression with high doses of proton pump inhibitors may result in partial or no regression of the BE. Medical treatment, however, does not appear to decrease incidence of adenocarcinoma. In a recent meta-analysis, in the medical group, there were 5.3 cancers per 1,000 patient-years. The only hope to improve the survival rate in these patients is to detect the cancer in an early and potentially curable stage.

One potential strategy to decrease mortality rate of adenocarcinoma is to identify patients at risk by screening patients, especially white men,50yearsor older with long-standing reflux by endoscopy with biopsy. The other way to decrease the incidence of lethal adenocarcinoma is endoscopic surveillance. Adenocarcinomas detected in a surveillance program are found at an earlier stage compared with patients not undergoing routine endoscopic surveillance. Indeed, a 5-year endoscopic surveillance program proved to be the most cost-effective strategy. Endoscopic surveillance, however, has not been evaluated in prospective randomized studies. The technique of surveillance is controversial: the number of biopsy samples, location of the biopsies, pathologic analysis, use of special stains, normal or jumbo biopsy forceps, etc. The intervals of surveillance are also under discussion; suggestions include 2–3 years without dysplasia,1yearwithlow grade dysplasia, and every3 months with high grade dysplasia.

## Ablation Therapy

Given the limitations of medical or surgical therapy, a variety of techniques of mucosal ablation have been evaluated based on the theory that after "burning" the abnormal (metaplastic and dysplastic) mucosa, squamous re-epithelization will occur in an environment with decreased or nonexistent acidity. The ablation can be accomplished by a variety of different techniques, such as thermal ablation, photodynamic therapy, and endoscopic mucosal resection.

Thermal ablation is performed by employing Nd:YAG laser or multipolar electro coagulation. Although there is histologic reversal in nearly 80% of patients, adverse effects have been described, such as chest pain, strictures, pleural effusion, and perforation. The follow up of patients is short, and there are some recurrences or maintenance of underlying intestinal metaplasia.

Photodynamic therapy utilizes a light-sensitive drug concentrated in neoplastic tissue. The drug is activated by light, producing toxicity which selectively injuries neoplastic tissues; it is a better therapy for long-segment BE. Although regression in several series varies from 70% to 90%, complete regression of BE is achieved in nearly 50% of patients. Intestinal metaplasia and even adenocarcinoma have been described, however, developing underneath the new squamous epithelium. Strictures may also occur.

These ablation therapies, although feasible, present a number of difficult issues, such as the persistence of intestinal metaplasia, development of adenocarcinoma in buried islands of intestinal metaplasia, and the eventual risks, costs, and maintenance of aggressive acid suppression therapy, either medical or surgical.

Endoscopic mucosal resection has become a potentially therapeutic procedure. It should be used in small(<20 mm), well-differentiated mucosal adenocarcinoma or high grade dysplasia. Complications can occur with subsequent development of high grade dysplasia or cancer. It is an alternative option in patients in whom the surgical risk is prohibitive.

# Medical Versus Surgical Therapy

DeMeester has defined the goals of management (medical or surgical) to be:

- To prevent the development of the metaplastic mucosa by stopping reflux early in the disease process.
- To promote or induce healing or regression of the metaplastic epithelium such that intestinal metaplasia is eliminated.
- To induce quiescence of the intestinalized metaplastic epithelium and halt its progression to dysplasia or cancer.

As has been discussed before, the goal of medical treatment of patients with BE is the control of symptoms; however, eradication of symptoms cannot be equated with elimination of reflux, and even after continuous medical treatment,

Barrett's mucosa develops in 12% of the patients. Furthermore, during continuous medical treatment, dysplasia and adenocarcinoma have appeared. Therefore, none of the three goals have been shown to be achieved adequately by medical treatment.

Several retrospective nonrandomized studies have compared medical and surgical treatment in patients with BE. Attwood performed a 3-year follow up in patients under medical treatment or who submitted to fundoplication, reporting better results after anti-reflux surgery. McCallum, Katz, and others suggested that anti-reflux surgery prevents the development of dysplasia and adenocarcinoma better than medical treatment.

There are three prospective, randomized studies concerning this aspect. Parrilla and colleagues in Spain found that symptomatic results were similar in both groups, but intestinal metaplasia did not disappear in any patient. There was persistence of acid reflux in 15% of the surgical patients. High grade dysplasia and adenocarcinoma appeared in a similar proportion in both groups. The important finding was that after successful anti-reflux surgery, results seem to be better than after medical treatment, although one patient in the surgical group also developed adenocarcinoma. Spechler also performed a prospective randomized study with a long followup. At 8–10 years after surgery, outcomes were similar, with the same proportion of patients in each group developing adenocarcinoma and nearly 65% of the surgical group needing antisecretory drugs. This study has seriously challenged the advantages of anti-reflux surgical treatment (fundoplication).

## Surgical Treatment

The goals of surgical treatment in patients with BE are outlined in Table 3.1. The results of patients with short-segment BE must be separated from those in patients with long-segment BE. From 1980 to 2005, some 32 articles addressed the surgical treatment of patients with BE, all involving classic

TABLE 3.1. Goals of surgical treatment in patients with Barrett's esophagus.

| | |
|---|---|
| 1. | Control of symptoms |
| 2. | To stop the reflux of acid and duodenal content to the distal esophagus |
| 3. | To prevent or eliminate the development of complications late after surgery, such as strictures |
| 4. | To prevent proximal progression to the BE |
| 5. | To induce regression of intestinal metaplasia to cardiac |
| 6. | To induce regression of dysplasia to non dysplastic muc |
| 7. | To prevent the progression towards dysplasia or adeno |

anti-reflux procedures, mainly Nissen fundoplication, Hill's posterior gastropexy, or Belsey Mark IV, Collis-Nissen, or Collis-Belsey procedures. Four publications addressed patients with short-segment BE. Unfortunately, as the final results are mixed with patients with long-segment BE, the only specific data are the loss of intestinal metaplasia and the eventual progression to dysplasia or adenocarcinoma. All four publications reported a certain degree of regression of intestinal metaplasia to cardiac mucosa but no progression to adenocarcinoma. Only one patient developed low grade dysplasia. Therefore, patients with short-segment BE can be treated by fundoplication, with very low morbidity or mortality and with good long term results.

In contrast, the results of anti-reflux surgery in patients with long-segment BE are as follows. Although the follow up is relatively short (80% have a follow up less than 5 years), there is an inverse correlation between clinical success and duration of follow up. The longer the follow up, poor outcomes and recurrence of reflux occur frequently due to the fact that acid reflux is not fully eliminated or stopped with antireflux surgery. In all reports in which there is mention of pH studies after surgery, positive values vary between 9% and 60%. Duodenal reflux has been evaluated in only two reports, and despite lack of symptomatic reflux, bile reflux may persist.

The effect of anti-reflux surgery in obtaining or achieving regression of intestinal metaplasia to cardiac or fundic mucosa in patients with long-segment BE has also been evaluated in 15 studies. Regression of intestinal metaplasia is rare (5%), and, therefore, operated patients require endoscopic surveillance. Classic anti-reflux surgery is unable to prevent development of adenocarcinoma, similar to results after medical treatment. Therefore, in patients with long-segment BE, classic anti-reflux surgery probably cannot be recommended as an anti-neoplastic measure, based on a meta-analysis.

In summary, although anti-reflux surgery effectively alleviates GERD symptoms in patients with long-segment BE, surgical outcome is less optimal, than that encountered in patients with GERD without BE. Complete regression of columnar mucosa is extremely uncommon, and long-term durability remains unanswered. Its role as a adjuvance to ablation therapy is unknown. Therefore, the reported results after anti-reflux surgery suggest that it does not influence markedly the natural history of BE concerning development of dysplasia or adenocarcinoma.

A surgical procedure that we have been using in patients with long-segment BE is the operation of acid suppression and duodenal diversion(Fig. 3.4). This procedure involves truncal or selective vagotomy, partial distal gastrectomy, fundoplication, and gastrojejunostomy with a Roux-en-Y limb 70 cm long. While ostensibly aggressive, acid production is decreased (vagotomy-gastrectomy), duodenal reflux is eliminated (Roux-en-Y drainage), and gastroesophageal reflux is diminished (fundoplication).

In patients with long-segment BE in whom there is a chronic and severe reflux not only of acid but also of duodenal content secondary to an incompetent LES, a significant dilation of the esophagogastric junction occurs in association with structural damage of the LES due to loss of the function of the clasp and sling fibers at this level. This phenomenon appears to explain why over long term follow up (10 years or more), the failure rate of classic anti-reflux surgery increases compared with the

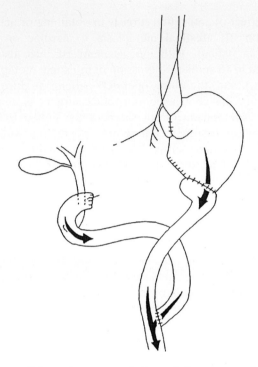

FIGURE 3.4. Schematic representation of the proposed surgical treatment for patients with long-segment Barrett's esophagus (Reprinted from Csendes, 2004).

results seen 2 or 3 years after surgery. We started to employ the technique of acid suppression and duodenal diversion in patients with long-segment BE. The results of 245 patients so treated are shown in Table 3.2. Symptoms of chronic reflux were controlled in 91%. Loss of intestinal metaplasia is 10 times greater when compared with classic anti-reflux surgery (55 vs. 5%). Regression of low grade dysplasia to non dysplastic mucosa is also greater. The most striking point is that after this operation, no adenocarcinoma has developed, and only 1% of patients have progressed to low grade dysplasia.

Our approach currently is the following. Patients with low grade dysplasia should undergo repeated endoscopy with

TABLE 3.2. Results of acid suppression and duodenal diversion, in patients with long-segment Barrett's esophagus ($n = 245$).

| | |
|---|---|
| Control of symptoms | 91% |
| Decrease of maximal acid output (PAO) | 90% |
| Percent patients with an abnormal (+) acid reflux | 15% |
| Percent patients with an abnormal (+) duodenal reflux | 5% |
| Regression of intestinal metaplasia to cardiac mucosa | 55% |
| Regression of low grade dysplasia to nondysplastic mucosa | 62% |
| Progression to dysplasia | 1% |
| Progression to adenocarcinoma | 0 |

1. Cardia intestinal metaplasia with symptoms and pathologic acid reflux
   ⟶         Laparoscopic antireflux surgery
2. Short-segment BE
   ⟶         Laparoscopic antireflux surgery
3. Complicated long segment BE
   ⟶         Laparoscopic antireflux surgery
   ⟶         Vagotomy-gastrectomy  with
             Roux-en-Y anastomosis + fundoplication
4. High grade dysplasia or adenocarcinoma
   ⟶         Esophagectomy

FIGURE 3.5. Proposed surgical treatment for patients with cardia intestinal metaplasia or Barrett's esophagus.

multiple biopsies. If pathologic review shows low grade dysplasia, the patient is treated with aggressive medical therapy for 1 year; if repeat endoscopy still shows low grade dysplasia and if functional studies (24 h pH monitoring and manometry) show that acid reflux is present, surgical therapy is suggested (Fig. 3.5). For the patient with short-segment BE and a negative Bilitec study (bile reflux), a laparoscopic Nissen fundoplication is performed. If the Bilitec study is positive or if the patient has a long-segment BE, our policy is to perform the more aggressive procedure of acid suppression and duodenal diversion. In 37 patients with low grade dysplasia submitted to this operation, regression of nondysplastic mucosa was obtained in 91%, while in patients with long-segment BE, this value was 63%.

The optimal treatment for patients with high-grade dysplasia is very controversial. DeMeester et al have proposed to treat this issue in a very precise and simple way:

- To determine the probability that adenocarcinoma will develop in a patient with high grade dysplasia over time.
- To determine the real value of all actual techniques to differentiate high grade dysplasia from adenocarcinoma.
- To determine which is the best option for treating these patients.

High-grade dysplasia will progress to adenocarcinoma in about 25% of patients followed for 2–3 years after diagnosis. Although high grade dysplasia without cancer follows a relatively benign course in the majority of patients, others develop cancer. A policy of endoscopic surveillance alone is not advisable, because adenocarcinoma even with lymph node metastasis can develop, and surgical results at that stage of disease should be considered.

Ablation therapy has been employed increasingly, and the results were discussed above. Two recent analyses addressing cost effectiveness of the different procedures in patients with high grade dysplasia have concluded that ablation therapy followed by endoscopic surveillance is a better option compared with esophagectomy, but these were theoretic analyses, and clinical trials should be performed in order to prove this approach.

For many patients, esophagectomy is the treatment of choice among those with high grade dysplasia and suspicion of adenocarcinoma. Obviously, it is mandatory to balance the potential risk of esophagectomy against the benefit of a curative resection. Therefore, esophagectomy should be performed only in a specialized surgical unit with a "high-volume" of esophageal operations. The procedure for restoration of the gastrointestinal tract can be either by colon interposition or a gastric pull up.

# Selected Readings

Csendes A (2004) Surgical treament of barrett's esohagus 1980-2003. World J Surg 28:225–231

Csendes A, Burdiles P, Braghetto I, Korn O (2004) Adeno-carcinoma appearing very late after antireflux surgery for Barrett's esophagus. Long term follow up, review of the literature and addition of six patients. J Gastrointest Surg 8:434–441

Csendes A, Burdiles P, Braghetto I, Smok G, Castro C, Korn O, Henriquez A (2002) Dysplasia and adenocarcinoma after classic antireflux surgery in patients with Barrett's esophagus. The need for long term subjective and objective follow up. Ann Surg 235:178–185

DeMeester TR (2001) Barrett's esophagus. Curr Probl Surg 38:549–640

Falk GW (2002) Barrett's esophagus. Gastroenterology 122:1569–1591

Nandurkar S, Talley NJ (1999) Barrett's esophagus: the long and the short of it. Am J Gastroent 94:30–40

Parrilla P, Martínez de Haro L, Ortiz A, et al. (2003) Long term results of a randomised prospective study comparing medical and surgical treatment of Barrett's esophagus. Ann Surg 237:291–298

Richter JE (2001) Antireflux surgery and adenocarcinoma of the esophagus. Let the truth be told. Gastroenterology 121:1506–1508

Spechler SJ (1997) The columnar lined esophagus. Gastrointest Clin N Am 26:455–466

# 4

# Achalasia: Chagas' Disease

**Ivan Cecconello, Flavio Roberto Takeda, and Henrique Walter Pinotti**

## Pearls and Pitfalls

- Chagas' disease is related etiologically to the protozoan hemoflagellate, *Trypanossoma cruzi* with destruction of Meissner's and Auerbach's plexuses of the esophagus.
- Esophagogram and manometry of the esophagus are fundamental for the diagnosis and allow classification into three stages: incipient, non-advanced, and advanced (end stage).
- Non-operative treatment provides only temporary relief of dysphagia.
- Cardiomyotomy with partial fundoplication is indicated in the non-advanced variant of achalasia and provides relief of dysphagia.
- Motility studies confirm a significant decrease of LES pressure after both types of operation, open or laparoscopic.
- The benefits of minimally invasive surgery include reduction of pain, short hospital stay, and more rapid return to normal activities.
- Advanced achalasia is treated by transhiatal esophagectomy without thoracotomy and cervical gastroplasty.
- The occurrence of Barrett's epithelium in the esophageal stump will prompt annual endoscopic follow-up and resection with disease progression.

K.I. Bland et al. (eds.), *Surgery of the Esophagus and Stomach*, DOI: 10.1007/978-1-84996-438-8_4, © Springer-Verlag London Limited 2011

- Construction of an elongated gastric tube (instead of the whole stomach) to achieve reduction in gastric acid and pepsin production with the continuous use of PPIs often proves of value with this challenge.
- Coloplasty should not be used due to the frequent association of achalasia and megacolon in Chagas' disease.

Chagas' disease is endemic and caused by the protozoan hemoflagellate, *Trypanossoma cruzi* and may affect multiple organs, particularly the myenteric plexus of the gastrointestinal tract and the heart. The involvement of the esophagus, including its dilatation, occurs in approximately 7–18% of patients in the chronic phases of Chagas' disease.

Different phases may be recognized in the history of chagasic achalasia: (1) occurrence of the disease in ancient South America was evident in pre-Inca and Inca mummies, (2) description of the clinical signs and symptoms of the disease and its geographic distribution (e.g., "choking disease" in Brazil) from the beginning of the 19th century to the first decades of the 20th century, (3) the period from the 2nd to the 7th decade of the 20th century when the morphologic and physiopathologic characteristics of the disease were defined, (4) recognition of the chagasicetiology of the diseases in the 1940s and 1950s, and (5) the current phase with evidence of a decrease in the incidence of the disease. Migration to urban areas, better sanitation, enhanced living conditions for the rural population, and the systematic application of insecticides to the residential dwellings are among principal factors responsible for control of the disease.

After the initial inoculation after a bite by the vector – a triatome which mixes its feces with the victim's blood - there is local growth of the trypanosoma. This phase is followed by a transient parasitemia (Fig. 4.1) lasting days or weeks, during which the microorganism lodges within various organs, notably, the gastrointestinal tract and the heart. The intensity of the parasitemia and the number of T. cruzi that infest different organs is dependent on an immunologic reaction between the parasite and the infected host.

In human Chagas' disease, there is a net loss of neurons from the autonomic system (Fig. 4.2). Early studies indicate

Figure 4.1. T. cruzi in a blood sample.

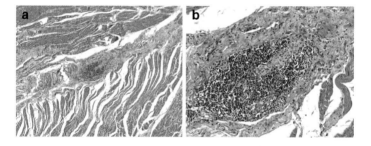

Figure 4.2. Inflammation of the myenteric plexus (**a**) with loss of esophageal ganglion cells (**b**) which were destroyed in the acute phase of disease in a patient with Chagasic achalasia.

that sera from over 80% of patients contained anti-neuron autoantibodies. Several groups have identified cross-reactive antibodies between T. cruzi and mammalian nervous tissue. A mononuclear inflammatory infiltrate occurs in the submucosal and muscular layer of esophageal wall with a net decrease of CD4 and T-cells and an inversion of the CD4/CD8 peripheral T-cell ratio.

*T. cruzi* infection may also function as a booster to autoimmunity and inflammatory cytokine production leading to tissue damage in individuals with susceptible genetic profiles.

With achalasia, the intensity of destruction of Meissner's and Auerbach's plexuses account for the subsequent pathophysiologic alterations and symptoms. It is believed that abnormality of motility (as detected by manometric methods) is found when >50% of these cells are destroyed; esophageal dilation occurs only when the destruction affects 90% of the ganglion cells. The major malfunctions detected by manometric studies are an achalasia-like hypertonicity of the lower esophageal sphincter (LES), aperistalsis, and swallowing waves of longer duration.

## Diagnosis

The major complaints of patients with achalasia are long-standing dysphagia and regurgitation frequently associated with nutritional depletion. Endoscopy of the upper digestive tract is essential to rule out the concomitant presence of carcinoma. Esophagography and manometry of the esophagus are fundamental for the diagnosis. These exams have enabled us to classify achalasia into three stages:

(a) *Incipient*: without esophageal dilation, but with specific motility disorders (achalasia-like changes and aperistalsis)
(b) *Non-advanced*: moderate dilation, stasis, and manometric findings of hyperactivity of the esophagus or aperistaltic waves with low amplitude and long duration
(c) *Advanced (end stage)*: frank dilation, atony of the body of the esophagus, or important megaesophagus (Fig. 4.3).

## Treatment

Nonoperative treatment of chagasic achalasia with drugs such as nifedipine has not produced consistent results; at most, these agents provide only temporary relief of

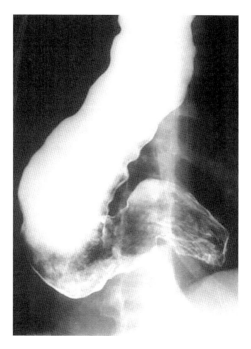

FIGURE 4.3. Esophagogram with an advanced disease—megaesophagus.

dysphagia. Botulin-toxin injection in the LES via endoscopy showed improvement of dysphagia in 58% of patients in a follow-up of 6 months; interestingly there was no significant decrease in the pressure of the LES after the intrasphincteric injection.

**Dilatation:** Hydrostatic dilation has been employed in many clinics with incipient achalasia. In a prospective randomized clinical study, 40 patients in the initial stage of achalasia managed by hydrostatic dilatation of the cardia (20 patients) or by cardiomyotomy with partial fundoplication (20 patients) were followed for3years. Both procedures were performed without substantial morbidity and no mortality. Results were similar regarding ongoing suppression of dysphagia. Radiologically, the methods were equivalent, because they promoted resolution of the stasis and maintenance of the esophageal diameter. Endoscopic follow-up did not show any differences between the procedures in terms of the development of reflux esophagitis, with a rate of only 5% for each group of patients. Manometry demonstrated that the operative treatment produced a greater decrease in LES sphincter pressure compared to manometric dilation, although the latter also decreased ES pressure. As measured by esophageal pH monitoring, dilatation demonstrated a greater propensity for reflux compared to the operative approach. It was concluded that both methods offer benefit in the treatment of the initial stage of achalasia; however, esophageal pH monitoring indicated that dilatation was associated with a greater index of esophageal acid exposition time.

**Cardiomyotomy with partial fundoplication** has been utilized in various clinics in the past 35 years. This technique combines a wide cardiomyotomy with a partial abdominal fundoplication. Initially patients were operated via an upper midline laparotomy; since 1991, the technique is via the laparoscopic approach. The procedure includes an extramucosal cardiomyotomy extending 2 cm below and 5–6 cm above the esophagogastric junction with mobilization of the gastric fundus and the "vasa breviae" when necessary. Thereafter, the superior surface of the fundus is sutured to the posterior esophageal wall followed by suturing to the anterior surface of the esophagus along the left and right margins of the myotomy (Fig. 4.4). Positioning of operative trocars is similar to that for the treatment of gastroesophageal reflux disease; any injury to the mucosa is sutured with monofilament 4-0 suture and is covered with the gastric fundus.

With this procedure, 1,029 patients were operated on by the authors through laparotomy and 297 with laparoscopic approach. Open surgery had a few intraoperative complications which included splenic injury (3%) corrected by electrocautery or by suturing, and mucosal perforation (4%). Mortality was <0.1% (Table 4.1).

In the patients operated on by laparoscopic approach (n = 297), mucosal perforation occurred in 4%, pleural lesions

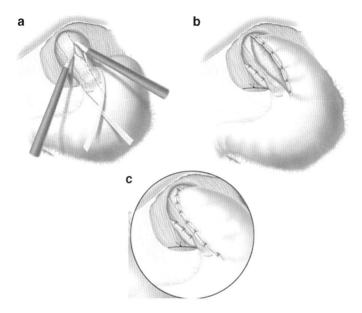

FIGURE 4.4. Surgical treatment of achalasia via a laparoscopic approach performing cardiomyotomy and fundoplication. (**a**) extramucosal cardiomyotomy; (**b**) the posterior surface of gastric fundus is sutured to the back of the esophageal wall and anterior surface of the esophagus along the left border of the myotomy; (**c**) final aspect after suture of the stomach to the right border of the myotomy.

TABLE 4.1. Cardiomyotomy and fundoplication complications.

|  | Open (%) n = 1029 | Laparoscopy (%) n = 297 |
|---|---|---|
| Splenic lesion | 3 | – |
| Splenectomy | 0.7 | – |
| Mucosa perforation | 4.4 | 4.4 |
| Pleural lesion | – | 0.7 |
| Esophageal fistulae | 0.02 | 0.3 |
| Pulmonary embolism | 0.01 | – |
| Mortality | 0.01 | 0.7 |
| Conversion to open operation |  | 1 |

in 1%, with three (1%) conversions to laparotomy. One patient had an esophageal fistula necessitating treatment by total parenteral nutrition. Mortality was 0.3% due to postoperative esophageal rupture secondary to regurgitation after feeding.

Relief of dysphagia was accomplished in most of the patients (Fig. 4.5). Motility studies confirmed a significant decrease of LES pressure after both types of operation. Decreases in the esophageal diameter were observed frequently after the procedure (Fig. 4.6). The benefits of minimally invasive approach include reduction in postoperative pain, shorter hospital stay, and faster return to normal activity.

**Associated diseases:** Additional (concomitant) involvement of the gastrointestinal tract by Chagas' disease with associated achalasia includes gastroparesis with impairment of gastric emptying, megaduodenum, and cholelithiasis. These conditions are treated concomitant with the achalasia, by pyloroplasty, latero-lateral duodenojejunostomy(with use of the third portion of the duodenum), and cholecystectomy.

When chagasic megacolon is evident, a mild degree of constipation can be treated with laxatives or with periodic rectal

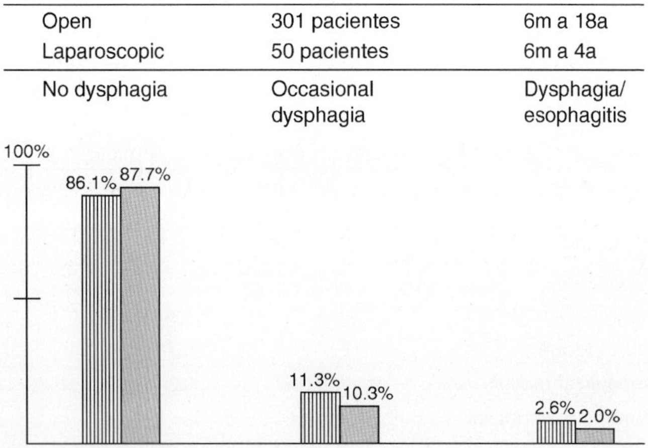

| Open | 301 pacientes | 6m a 18a |
| Laparoscopic | 50 pacientes | 6m a 4a |
| No dysphagia | Occasional dysphagia | Dysphagia/ esophagitis |

100%

86.1% 87.7%

11.3% 10.3%

2.6% 2.0%

FIGURE 4.5. Late follow-up results in patients submitted to cardiomyotomy and partial fundoplication.

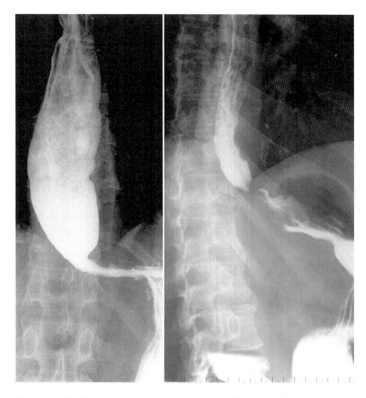

FIGURE 4.6. Esophagogram of a patient with achalasia before and after cardiomyotomy and partial fundoplication.

enemas. Patients with intractable and recurrent fecal impaction or recurrent sigmoid volvulus must be treated surgically. On rare occasion, the disorder is treated simultaneously with achalasia. In our experience, the treatment of choice is rectosigmoidectomy with immediate, posterior, end-to-side colorectostomy.

**Esophagectomy without thoracotomy:** In order to avoid thoracotomy and blind dissection, a technique for removing the esophagus under direct vision with wide opening of the diaphragm through the abdominal route was developed by Pinotti and includes:

- Upper median laparotomy with phrenotomy (Figs. 4.7a and b);
- Retraction of the pericardium and pleura with cranial dissection of the esophagus. Special types of cauterization and/or clipping can be used for ligating vessels around the esophagus or arising from the aorta
- A second team approaches the cervical esophagus simultaneously via a left transverse cervical incision, 2 cm above the left clavicle. The esophagus is freed distally with special retractors and transected at the level chosen for the anastomosis
- After complete dissection, the esophagus is removed through the abdominal incision
- The stomach is freed preserving the right vascular pedicles and part of the lesser curvature is resected with the esophagus (Fig. 4.7c)
- The stomach is pulled up through the posterior mediastinum and anastomosed to the cervical esophagus (Fig. 4.7d)

Postoperative enteral feeding is maintained for 10 days until radiologic demonstration of an intact anastomosis. Enteral feeding can be prolonged during the period of closure of any eventual anastomotic fistula.

One hundred and sixty-six patients with advanced achalasia were operated utilizing the described technique. The mortality rate for the series was 3.0%. Deaths were attributable to fistulas related to the pyloroplasty, mediastinal hemorrhage, and acute pancreatitis in the immediate postoperative period. Eighty-three patients were followed for an average time of 8 years (3–27 years). All underwent clinical and endoscopic evaluation pre-and post-operatively at 6 months ( Table 4.2). Dumping and diarrhea occurred primarily early after operation due to the vagotomy during the esophagectomy.

All patients treated with esophagectomy without thoracotomy returned to social life and were able to join the work force; mild dysphagia was observed in 6% of the patients. Weight gain was observed in 80%. One patient developed a squamous cell carcinoma in the esophageal stump 13 years after esophagectomy which was resected locally.

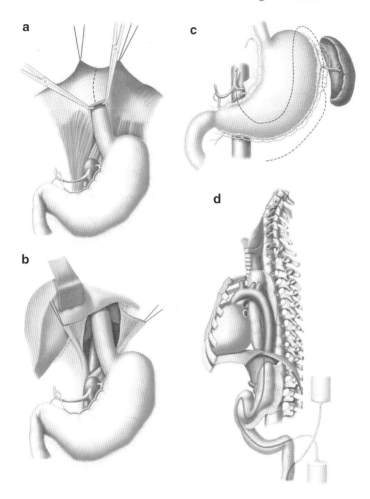

FIGURE 4.7. Surgical treatment of advanced achalasia through esophagectomy without thoracotomy. (**a**) Upper laparotomy with median phrenotomy; (**b**) dissection of the esophagus through the lower mediastinum; (**c**) mobilization of the stomach; d pull-up of the stomach to the cervical region with esophagogastric anastomosis.

Clinical and endoscopic findings confirmed a clinically important increase in heartburn, regurgitation, diffuse gastritis, esophagitis, and Barrett's epithelium in the esophageal

TABLE 4.2. Esophagectomy without thoracotomy: late follow-up (83 patients).

|  | 6 m (%) | 7 years (%) |
|---|---|---|
| Dysphagia | 30 | 6 |
| Regurgitation | 34 | 35 |
| Heartburn | 12 | 45 |
| Weight gain | 71 | 76 |
| Diarrhea | 44 | 2 |
| Dumping | 15 | 1 |
| Esophagitis | 20 | 66 |
| Barrett esophagus | – | 27 |

stump with time due to duodeno-gastroesophageal reflux. Continuous use of PPIs (proton-pump inhibitors) was suggested. The presence of Barrett's epithelium in the esophageal stump demands annual endoscopic and histologic follow-up. Employment of an elongated gastric tube (instead of the whole stomach) in order to decrease gastric acid and pepsin production may be of value in this challenge.

Esophagectomy with cervical esophagogastrostomy remains an excellent choice for the treatment of end-stage chagasic achalasia. Due to the possible occurrence of simultaneous megacolon, coloplasty is not recommended.

## Selected Readings

Bettarello A, Pinotti HW (1976) Oesophageal involvement in Chagas' disease. Clin Gastroenterol 5:103–117

Cecconello I (1998) Long-term evaluation of gastroplasty in achalasia. In: Siewert R, Holsher AH (eds) Diseases of the esophagus. Springer-Verlag, Berlin, pp. 975–978

Cecconello I, Marianoda Rocha J, Zilberstein B et al. (1993) Reflux esophagitis and development of ectopic columnar epithelium in the esophageal stump after gastric transposition. In: Nabeia K, Hanaoka T, Nogami T (eds) Recent advances in diseases of the esophagus. Springer-Verlag, Berlin

Cunha-Neto E (2001) Understanding the immunopathogenesis of Chagas disease: perspectives for the new millennium. In: Pinotti HW, Cecconello I, Felix VN, Oliveira MA (eds) Recent advances in disease of the esophagus. Manduzzi Editore, Bologna, pp. 197–204 da Silveira AB, Arantes RM, Vago AR et al. (2005) Comparative study of the presence of Trypanosoma cruzi kDNA, inflammation and denervation in chagasic patients with and without megaesophagus. Parasitology 131:627–634

Felix VN (1998) Achalasia: a prospective results of dilatation and myotomy. Hepatogastroenterol 45:97–108

Meneguelli UF (2001) Chagasic megaesophagus - historical aspects and present situation in South America. In: Pinotti HW, Cecconello I, Felix VN, Oliveira MA (eds) Recent advances in disease of the esophagus. Manduzzi Editore, Bologna, pp. 197–204

Moraes-Filho JP, Bettarello A (1989) Response of the lower esophageal sphincter to pentagastrin on patients with megaesophagus secondary to Chagas' disease. Rev Hosp Clin Fac Med Sao Paulo 44:178–180

Pinotti HW (1964) Contribuicão para o estudo de fisiopa-tologia do megaesôfago. Thesis, Faculdade de Medicina da Universidade de São Paulo

Pinotti HW. (1988) The basis of its treatment. In: Siewert JR, Holscher AH (eds) Diseases of esophagus. Springer-Verlag, Berlin, pp. 17–19

# 5
# Esophageal Perforation

**S. Michael Griffin and Jonathan Shenfine**

## Pearls and Pitfalls

- Esophageal perforation is a rare but hazardous event.
- Iatrogenic damage during upper gastrointestinal endoscopy accounts for the majority of injuries.
- Therapeutic endoscopy carries a 200-fold higher perforation risk than diagnostic endoscopy.
- Clinical features depend on the cause, site and time of injury.
- Severe, sudden chest pain after vomiting associated with subcutaneous emphysema is pathognomic of spontaneous perforation of the esophagus.
- Survival is dependent on rapid control of mediastinal and pleural contamination.
- Surgery is mandatory when gross contamination is present, when there is tissue loss or in perforations associated with caustic injuries.
- Thorough wound debridement, lavage of pleural and mediastinal cavities and drainage are probably more important than any specific repair technique employed in cases where surgery is performed.

## Introduction

Esophageal perforation is a rare event, which can occur through a variety of insults and carries a high morbidity and mortality due to difficulty in accessing the esophagus, the

K.I. Bland et al. (eds.), *Surgery of the Esophagus and Stomach*, DOI: 10.1007/978-1-84996-438-8_5, © Springer-Verlag London Limited 2011

unusual blood supply, the lack of a strong serosal layer, and the proximity of vital structures. The limited exposure that clinicians gain often means that few have the knowledge and skills required to deal with these injuries. This lack of experience is compounded by the lack of an evidence base for management, which is directly due to the scarcity of cases and heterogeneous presenting features. As a result, misdiagnosis and inappropriate management are all too common with potentially catastrophic consequences.

This chapter focuses on the diagnosis and management of spontaneous and iatrogenic esophageal perforation, external trauma and caustic perforation.

# Etiology

## *Iatrogenic Perforation of the Esophagus*

Iatrogenic damage to the esophagus can occur from within, such as during endoscopic instrumentation, or from without such as by paraesophageal surgery, with the former being far more common. Due to advances in imaging technology and the inherent safety of the procedure with a relatively low risk of esophageal perforation (0.03% of diagnostic procedures), flexible videoendoscopy has almost totally replaced rigid esophagoscopy. However, despite this safety record, a dramatic increase in the number of endoscopic examinations performed and associated instrumentation has led to a rise in the number of iatrogenic injuries with an associated overall mortality rate of 19%. As such, prevention of these injuries by awareness and training is most likely to reduce the rate of morbidity and mortality.

Inappropriate force used to "intubate" the esophagus can easily cause a proximal perforation and this hazard is augmented with hyper-extension of the neck, arthritis of the cervical spine or in the presence of an esophageal diverticulum. However, by far the majority (75–90%) of iatrogenic perforations occur in the distal esophagus often in the presence of an underlying abnormality, such as a benign or malignant stricture, with perforation occurring just above due to formation of a false passage or from within due to splitting of the abnormal esophagus. Therapeutic endoscopy carries a 200-fold higher perforation risk (approximately 5%) than diagnostic endoscopy, both for cancer-related procedures and those carried out for benign conditions. Endoscopic palliation of malignant dysphagia especially where pre-dilatation of malignant strictures has been used accounts for the majority of injuries. The risk is greatest in patients who have received prior radiotherapy or chemotherapy. Pneumatic dilatation for achalasia remains a high-risk procedure due to the high pressures and large diameter balloon involved. Perforation is also possible with variceal ligation and sclerotherapy and these procedures may be associated with delayed perforation due to transmural necrosis.

Non-endoscopic instrumentation of the esophagus can also lead to direct trauma, for example, from nasogastric tube or transesophageal echocardiography probe insertion. It can also be due to from esophageal intubation by an endotracheal tube or indirect trauma from pressure necrosis due to the cuff of a tracheal tube or, even from close lying intercostal chest drains. Paraesophageal surgery, such as anti-reflux surgery, can also inadvertently lead to direct trauma, but the risk is low (0–1.2%).

## Spontaneous Perforation of the Esophagus

The rare, eponymous Boerhaave's syndrome is defined as complete disruption of the esophageal wall occurring in the absence of pre-existing pathology. It is characterized by barogenic esophageal injury leading to immediate and gross gastric content contamination of the pleural cavity, with rapid and catastrophic onset of chemical and bacterial mediastinitis. A history of a sudden rise in intra-abdominal pressure is present in 80–90% of cases usually as a result of retching or vomiting but cases have resulted from blunt trauma, weight lifting, parturition, defecation, the Heimlich maneuver or status epilepticus.

Vomiting results from involuntary abdominal and dia-phragmatic contraction with pyloric closure and cricopharyn-geus relaxation, and raised intra-abdominal pressure leading to reflux of gastric contents through a passive esophagus. Mackler demonstrated in the 1950s that if flow is obstructed, then an increase in intra-luminal pressure suddenly occurs, and a rapid rise of only 5 psi can result in esophageal perfora-tion. However, although vomiting is commonplace, spontane-ous perforation of the esophagus is so rare factors that are as yet undetermined, may be of relevance.

## Penetrating Injuries of the Esophagus

Sharp, penetrating injuries of the thoracic esophagus are uncommon except with gunshot wounds but the more superficially lying cervical esophagus may be injured by knife wounds to the neck. These injuries often occur in conjunction with other serious injuries to surrounding vis-cera so are easily missed and the consequent delay greatly increases morbidity and mortality. A high index of suspicion, based on the tract of the injury is therefore of paramount importance.

## Blunt Esophageal Trauma

Blunt esophageal trauma is extremely uncommon and usu-ally occurs only in conjunction with high velocity injuries. As such, they are often associated with immediately life threat-ening airway or cardiopulmonary damage and compromise. In rapid deceleration events, the otherwise well protected thoracic esophagus may be injured by traction laceration, vascular thrombosis or barogenic damage. Blunt cervical esophageal perforation can occur when the neck or upper chest impacts a fixed structure, by extreme "whiplash" flex-ion-extension or an associated cervical fracture — usually in cases from road traffic accidents.

## Caustic Injuries

Serious ingestion of a caustic substance leading to esophageal perforation is uncommon but devastating. Although accidental ingestion in childhood account for the majority of caustic trauma injuries, adult ingestion are more often deliberate with suicidal intent and are therefore usually the more serious in nature. Most caustic substances can be grouped into acids or alkalis and are readily available as cleaners, in batteries and in industrial practice. Acids are unpleasant to swallow and produce a coagulative necrosis and are thus less likely to be penetrative. In contrast, alkalis are marginally more palatable and resultant liquefactive necrosis is rapidly transmural. However, in general, the severity of the injury is related to the concentration, amount, viscosity, and duration of contact between the caustic agent and the esophageal mucosa and the ingestion of any strong caustic agent in sufficient quantity will inflict a potentially fatal esophageal injury.

# Clinical Presentation

Clinical features of esophageal perforation depend on the cause, site and duration after injury.

Full-thickness, intrathoracic, iatrogenic perforations are usually recognized and visualized immediately or there is at least a high index of suspicion. They are commonly associated with chest pain, dysphagia and odynophagia, often allied to a sympathetic nervous system response with pallor, sweating, peripheral circulatory shutdown, tachycardia, tachypnea and overt hemodynamic shock. Systemic symptoms are less common with cervical perforations which present with neck pain, dysphonia, cervical dysphagia, hoarseness, and subcutaneous emphysema predominating.

Spontaneous esophageal perforation classically presents with sudden, distressing, retrosternal or epigastric pain following an episode of raised intra-abdominal pressure, usually vomiting, with subsequent subcutaneous emphysema (Mackler's triad). A dramatic sympathetic nervous system response is usually present. Within 24–48 h a systemic inflammatory response gives way to cardiopulmonary collapse and multiorgan failure as a consequence of overwhelming bacterial mediastinitis.

Penetrating esophageal trauma manifests in the same fashion as iatrogenic trauma but a high index of suspicion, based on the tract of the injury is essential for diagnosis; damage should be suspected in any transcervical or transmediastinal wound, especially when gunshot derived.

Blunt esophageal trauma is rare and usually only occurs in high impact events so is frequently associated with more immediately life threatening airway or cardiopulmonary damage. Again a high index of suspicion is necessary and esophageal perforation actively excluded.

Clinical features in patients with caustic esophageal perforation are dependent on the substance and the time course since ingestion. The absence of oral burns or pharyngo-esophageal symptoms does not exclude a significant esophageal injury. However, drooling and hypersalivation are common when oropharyngeal burns are present and together with stridor and hoarseness are the warning signs of potentially life-threatening airway edema. The typical symptoms of esophageal injury are of dysphagia and odynophagia and perforation should be suspected with severe retrosternal or epigastric pain especially if this radiates to the back, and is accompanied by abdominal tenderness, shock, respiratory distress, pleural pain, or subcutaneous emphysema. In contrast to other injuries, a perforation may develop as a delayed phenomenon and intensive observation and re-assessment of these patients is vital.

## Investigations

A classical history and thus a high clinical suspicion is the most reliable parameter for the successful diagnosis of esophageal perforation, but atypical symptoms, the similarity to more common cardiorespiratory disorders and a shocked, confused and distressed patient can misdirect the clinician. As time passes, the critical condition of the patient obscures relevant clinical features and the pursuit of incorrect investigations make the diagnosis even more elusive. The following investigations are the most helpful in establishing the diagnosis.

## Plain Radiography

The typical findings of esophageal perforation on a plain chest radiograph are pleural effusion, pneumomediastinum, subcutaneous emphysema, hydropneumothorax, pneumothorax and collapse or consolidation but these findings may be subtle and are dependent on the site, the extent of trauma and the time interval following the insult. Figure 5.1 demonstrates the typical

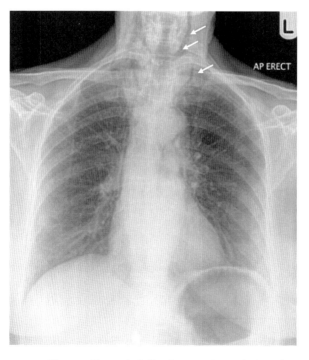

FIGURE 5.1. Chest radiograph following esophageal dilatation of a benign stricture demonstrating pneumomediastinum (arrows highlight gas in the left mediastinum).

appearance of an esophageal perforation causing pneumomediastinum following the dilatation of a benign stricture. In
caustic injuries there may be radiographic signs of aspiration.

## Contrast Radiography

Oral water soluble contrast radiography (Fig. 5.2) is the
investigation of choice to confirm perforation and this helps

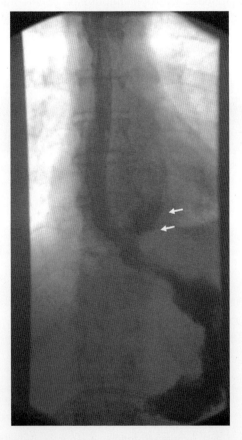

FIGURE 5.2. Contrast swallow demonstrating esophageal leak.
A naso-jejunal feeding tube has been sited.

to ascertain the site, degree of containment and degree of drainage and aqueous agents are rapidly absorbed, do not exacerbate inflammation and have minimal tissue effects. False negative results are not uncommon with contrast studies due to the rapid passage of low-viscosity contrast past a small hole closed by edema or due to extravasation of contrast from the tear site parallel to the esophageal shadow. As such, if negative, films should be repeated in the lateral or oblique positions or using barium.

## Upper Gastrointestinal Endoscopy

Flexible videoendoscopy is an expert procedure as it carries significant risk in inexperienced hands. Figure 5.3 demonstrates the endoscopic appearance of a spontaneous esophageal perforation. Nevertheless, with fluoroscopic guidance it allows crucial assessment of the site, the mucosal trauma, and reveals any underlying pathology facilitating placement of a nasogastric or nasojejunal tube for drainage or feeding. This is especially useful in an "on table" situation where trauma is suspected but

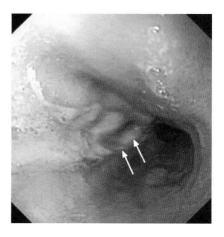

FIGURE 5.3. Endoscopic view of spontaneous esophageal perforation.

where other injuries preclude radiological examination. Similarly, in caustic injuries, endoscopy allows assessment of the stomach for possible reconstruction.

## Computed Tomography (CT)

CT is an increasingly useful investigation (Fig. 5.4) in those patients stable enough to undergo scanning but the radiology department is a dangerous place for an unstable patient. CT is especially useful in cases of external trauma, caustic injuries and in critically ill patients with an atypical presentation. In combination with interventional radiological techniques, CT has also revolutionized the management of intra-thoracic collections.

## Other

Drainage of gastric contents on thoracocentesis is diagnostic and may be aided by measurement of pH, amylase or microscopy for squamous cells. Administration of oral dyes, such as

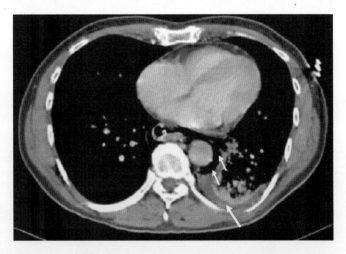

FIGURE 5.4. CT chest demonstrating pneumomediastinum and contamination of left pleural cavity.

methylene blue, may be a useful adjunct if there is a communicating drain.

# Management

All patients with esophageal perforation should be viewed as critically ill. The immediate priorities are the establishment of a secure and adequate airway, the stabilization of cardiovascular status and the relief of pain. The initial resuscitation is documented in Table 5.1 and regular re-assessment is obligatory.

The rarity of esophageal injuries and the consequences of incorrect management have limited the ability to evaluate differing treatments. Published case series often span

TABLE 5.1. Initial resuscitation following suspected esophageal perforation.

| Initial resuscitation |
|---|
| Control of airway |
| Administration of oxygen |
| Early anesthetic assessment |
| Large bore intravenous access |
| Intravenous fluid resuscitation |
| Central venous access and arterial line monitoring. inotropic support |
| Urethral catheterization |
| Fluid balance monitoring |
| Intravenous broad spectrum antibiotic and antifungal agents |
| Intravenous antisecretory agents (proton pump inhibitors) |
| Strict nil by mouth |
| Large bore intercostal chest drainage   possibly bilaterally |
| Nasogastric tube (only to be placed under endoscopic vision or radiological guidance) |

many years, many centers, many surgeons and many techniques. Non-operative treatment has become the standard management of iatrogenic esophageal perforation with a low mortality due to sophisticated respiratory, nutritional and antimicrobial support but this should be viewed as "radical" in other situations. Survival is dependent on avoiding or controlling mediastinal and pleural contamination and surgery remains mandatory when gross contamination is present, and there is loss of tissue or when the perforation has been due to a caustic injury. Where possible, all patients with an esophageal perforation should be managed in specialist units by specialist surgeons with a multi-disciplinary approach to care. Hospitals lacking in these specialist facilities or the appropriate and versatile surgical cover necessary to operate on the esophagus by abdominal or left or right thoracic approaches, should transfer the patients at the earliest opportunity after stabilization.

## Non-operative Management

With advances in radiological interventional techniques, antibiotics and enteral nutrition, successful non-operative management is possible in selected patients. Two patient groups in particular are suitable for consideration: those diagnosed rapidly with minimal contamination or those with a delayed diagnosis who have demonstrated tolerance to the perforation. Some guidance for patient selection is possible using the criteria detailed in Table 5.2.

## Distal Perforation

Patients require intensive observation and should strictly not receive any oral intake. Chest drains are placed where pleural perforation has occurred and contrast radiology, endoscopy and CT performed to monitor the status of the esophageal

Table 5.2. Criteria for non-operative management of esophageal perforation.

| Criteria for non-operative management of esophageal perforation |
| --- |
| Contained perforation |
| Free flow of contrast back into esophagus on contrast swallow |
| No symptoms or signs of mediastinitis |
| No evidence of solid food contamination of pleural or mediastinal cavities |
| **Other factors to consider** |
| Perforation is "controlled" |
| No underlying esophageal disease or loss of tissue |
| Non-caustic injury |
| No sepsis |
| Availability for intensive observation and access to multi-disciplinary care |
| Low threshold for intervention |
| Enteral feeding established |

leak and collections. All patients should be given broad-spectrum, intravenous antibiotics, anti-fungal and anti-secretory agents with a low threshold for drainage of collections and surgical intervention. Enteral feeding may be established using a surgical feeding jejunostomy or a naso-jejunal feeding tube placed under endoscopic and/or radiological assistance together with a nasogastric tube placed to decompress the stomach. Non-operative treatment must not be "conservative" and intervention when required, should be rapid and aggressive.

Removable self-expanding metal stents may help to seal iatrogenic perforations of malignant tumors if deemed unfit for resection but stent insertion cannot be recommended for perforations within a normal esophagus, as expansion of the stent may expand the defect.

## Cervical Perforation

Perforations of the cervical esophagus are often managed non-operatively with percutaneous drainage of collections. However, when uncontained, primary closure with prevertebral lavage and drainage using a left lateral incision anterior to the sternocleidomastoid is recommended and is tolerated well by even critically ill patients.

## Operative Management

Surgery is appropriate if the patient has overt signs of sepsis, shock, gross contamination, an underlying obstructive pathology, a retained foreign body, a caustic injury or has failed non-operative management. Virtually all gunshot wounds require surgery. The prime objectives are to clear the contamination and then to restore esophageal integrity whilst preventing further soiling. A feeding jejunostomy should be fashioned for enteral feeding. Depending on the perforation site, a right sided (for upper or mid esophagus) or left sided (distal esophagus) postero-lateral thoracotomy is used at an appropriate level. The pleural cavity is cleaned and lavaged, the mediastinal pleura incised to expose the injury and necrotic, and devitalized tissue debrided. In spontaneous perforation, an extended myotomy should be made as the mucosal injury is usually longer than the muscular one. Iatrogenic perforations frequently occur in association with an underlying pathology such as carcinoma, peptic stricture or achalasia. As a result, surgery can have a high mortality rate despite minimal contamination.

## Primary Repair

A primary suture repair is the most common surgical technique and may be buttressed with nearby tissues to reinforce the suture line. This repair is associated with a high leak rate so should be reserved for those with demonstrably healthy tissue and limited soiling.

Repair over a T-tube is a viable alternative in view of the high leak rate for primary repair. This diverts swallowed secretions via a controlled esophago-cutaneous fistula allowing healing to occur without ongoing contamination. A 6–10 mm diameter T-tube is placed through the tear with the limbs directed proximally and distally beyond the boundaries of the perforation and the esophageal wall is closed around loosely. The tube is brought out through the chest wall and secured with a further drain placed down to the repair and apical and basal intercostal chest drains. The T-tube is left until a defined tract is established with the majority removed between 3 and 6 weeks.

## Exclusion and Diversion

Exclusion of the contaminated mediastinum and diversion of secretions maximizes healing while minimizing risk. Although the techniques used to achieve this are complex and do not appear to achieve any better results than other simpler treatments, it remains in the armamentarium of the esophageal surgeon.

## Resection

Esophageal resection is a major undertaking, but in the presence of a diseased esophagus, may be the only solution. Immediate reconstruction can be employed where there is minimal contamination but a delayed approach can also be adopted. Patients with a caustic perforation almost always require an emergency esophago-gastrectomy as the stomach is also usually injured. Immediate reconstruction with a colonic interposition graft can be performed or delayed for 6–8 weeks if there is minimal local contamination. Resection should also be considered in patients with extensive, circumferential mucosal injuries as these can lead to problematic strictures and a significant long term cancer risk. An alternative, if the esophagus is intact and respiratory complications supervene, is defunctioning via a cervical esophagostomy and the formation of a feeding jejunostomy with resection and reconstruction delayed until the patient is stable. The mortality for these injuries is between 13% and 40% with the majority of deaths occurring in the adult suicidal group. Mortality mainly stems from respiratory complications and delay in aggressive surgical treatment of transmural necrosis. There is no place for "conservative" treatment in the case of a severe caustic injury.

## Perforation and Cancer

Perforation of an inoperable malignant stricture should be managed non-operatively, in this situation a sealing self-expanding metal stent may be the most appropriate treatment. In patients with less clearly defined operability most authors recommend resection. However, this carries considerably mortality (between 22 and 75%) and long term survival is compromised such that this treatment should be considered palliative. As such, every effort should be made to prevent iatrogenic injury during staging procedures.

## Conclusions

The fragility of the esophageal wall, the lack of serosa, the proximity of vital organs, the inaccessibility and the lack of symptoms and signs can mean that even small perforations of the esophagus can be ultimately fatal. Overall mortality for esophageal perforation from any cause is high and the majority of surgeons only deal with a handful of difficult cases in their career. These cases are therefore best managed by specialist units with ancillary staff trained, equipped and experienced to prevent the potentially disastrous consequences of misdiagnosis and inappropriate management. Prevention of iatrogenic injuries through appropriate endoscopic training is the key to improving outcomes.

# Selected Readings

Abbott OA, Mansour KA, Logan WD Jr et al. (1970) Atraumatic so-called "spontaneous" rupture of the esophagus. A review of 47 personal cases with comments on a new method of surgical therapy. J Thorac Cardiovasc Surg 59:67–83

Bufkin BL, Miller JI Jr, Mansour KA (1996) Esophageal perforation: emphasis on management. Ann Thorac Surg 61:1447–1451; discussion 51–2

Derbes VJ, Mitchell RE Jr (1955) Hermann Boerhaave's Atrocis, nec descripti prius, morbi historia, the first trans-lation of the classic case report of rupture of the esophagus, with annotations. Bull Med Libr Assoc 43:217–240

Estrera A, Taylor W, Mills LJ et al. (1986) Corrosive burns of the esophagus and stomach: a recommendation for an aggressive surgical approach. Ann Thorac Surg 41:276–283

Griffin SM, Lamb PJ, Shenfine J et al. (2008) Spontaneous rupture of the oesophagus. Br J Surg 95:1432–1439

Jones WG 2nd, Ginsberg RJ (1992) Esophageal perforation: a continuing challenge. Ann Thorac Surg 53:534–543

Mackler S (1952) Spontaneous rupture of the esophagus: an experimental and clinical study. Surg Gynecol Obstet 95:345–356

Zargar SA, Kochhar R, Nagi B et al. (1992) Ingestion of strong corrosive alkalis: spectrum of injury to upper gastrointestinal tract and natural history. Am J Gastroenterol 87:337–341

# 6
# Esophageal Diverticula

**Jörg Hutter and Hubert J. Stein**

## Pearls and Pitfalls

- Only symptomatic esophageal diverticula require treatment
- Most traction diverticula are asymptomatic
- Pulsion diverticula are due to a distal functional esophageal obstruction (motor disorder)
- Surgical treatment must address the underlying pathogenetic mechanism, i.e. a myotomy at the site of the functional distal obstruction in pulsion diverticula is mandatory
- Minimally invasive (endoscopic, thoracoscopic, laparoscopic) approaches are feasible but still associated with high complication or failure rates

## Introduction

A diverticulum is a pouch or sac that protrudes from the gastrointestinal wall and can derive from any tubular organ in the gastrointestinal tract. True diverticula contain all layers of the gastrointestinal wall. Most diverticula of the esophagus consist of mucosa, submucosa, and strands of muscle fibers only and are, therefore, "false" diverticula.

K.I. Bland et al. (eds.), *Surgery of the Esophagus and Stomach*, DOI: 10.1007/978-1-84996-438-8_6,
© Springer-Verlag London Limited 2011

Esophageal diverticula are classified according to their location (cervical vs. midesophageal vs. epiphrenic) and the presumed underlying pathogenetic mechanism (pulsion vs. traction). Pulsion diverticula typically occur proximal to a physiologic sphincter or proximal to areas of functional resistance to food passage and are assumed to be caused by excessive intraluminal pressure on the esophageal wall. Traction diverticula result from traction forces arising from outside the esophageal wall and usually occur in response to periesophageal inflammation such as chronic lymphadenitis.

The most common diverticula in the upper digestive tract are Zenker's diverticula. They are located in the cervical region and originate from the posterior wall of the hypopharynx proximal to the upper esophageal sphincter. These esophageal diverticula should, thus, be more adequately termed hypopharyngeal diverticula. Midesophageal diverticula are those at or close to the level of the tracheal bifurcation while epiphrenic diverticula are located within a few centimeters proximal to the lower esophageal sphincter (Fig. 6.1).

## Zenker's Diverticulum

A Zenker's diverticulum results from an outpouching in a weak muscular portion at the posterior hypopharyngeal wall immediately proximal to the upper esophageal sphincter, the so-called Killian's triangle. They are diagnosed typically in persons over the age of 50 years and are more common in males than females. The estimated incidence is 2 per 100,000/year.

The pathogenesis of Zenker's diverticulum is related to a decreased compliance of the cricopharyngeal muscle, the major component of the upper esophageal sphincter. This decreased compliance results in decreased contractility and increased resistance to the passage of a bolus from the hypopharynx into the cervical esophagus. The most widely accepted pathogenic mechanism of these diverticula is related to a dysfunction of the upper esophageal sphincter, e.g. abnormal or inadequate opening of the upper esophageal sphincter on

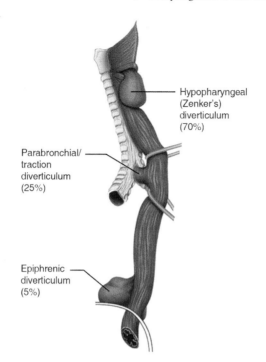

Hypopharyngeal
(Zenker's)
diverticulum
(70%)

Parabronchial/
traction
diverticulum
(25%)

Epiphrenic
diverticulum
(5%)

FIGURE 6.1. Typical location and frequency distribution of esophageal diverticular (Modified from Stein et al., 2006. With permission of Springer Science and Business Media).

swallowing as a result of a primary myogenic or neurologic disorder. This theory is supported by the observation of an increased intrabolus pressure on hypopharngeal manometry in patients with Zenker's diverticulum. Whether chronic gastroesophageal reflux can also contribute to the formation of a Zenker's diverticulum is still controversial.

Over time, a permanent, narrow-mouthed outpouching of the posterior hypopharyngeal wall develops and enlarges inevitably. As a result, saliva, secretions, liquid, and food will pool dependently in the diverticulum sac and cannot empty easily into the esophagus. In the early phase, patients may complain only of a vague globus sensation, intermittent cough, and excessive salivation. Intermittent dysphagia, regurgitation of undigested foods, and aspiration follow as the disease and the size of the diverticulum progress. A Zenker's diverticulum may become large enough to produce a visible mass in the neck, which may gurgle on palpation (Boyce's sign) or obstruct the esophagus by compression. To aid in swallowing, patients may develop elaborate maneuvers: clearing the throat, coughing, or placing external pressure on the neck. The most serious complication associated with Zenker's diverticulum is aspiration, which can lead to pneumonia or lung abscess. Perforation (sometimes iatrogenic on forceful attempts to access the esophagus with an endoscope or a tube), bleeding, and carcinoma may also complicate Zenker's diverticula.

Small Zenker's diverticula are often missed on endoscopy. Thus, endoscopy is not the method of choice to establish a diagnosis, but it is often used to exclude other upper gastrointestinal disorders. Usually, a Zenker's diverticulum is diagnosed with contrast radiography. Small diverticula can be missed if they are superimposed on the main column of barium in the esophagus. This error can be avoided by rotating the patient during the examination and using high speed video or cinematographic recordings of the pharyngoesophageal phase of swallowing (Fig. 6.2). Esophageal manometry is not required typically; however, it may help to illuminate the functional obstruction at the upper esophageal sphincter and the increased intrabolus pressure in the hypopharyngeal region.

Every symptomatic Zenker's diverticulum, irrespective of its size, is considered an indication for operative intervention. Based on its pathogenesis, the treatment of Zenker's diverticulum is aimed at the underlying disorder of the upper esophageal sphincter with the goal of increasing the compliance of the upper esophageal sphincter and facilitating its opening during a swallow. Standard operative treatment, thus, comprises a simple cricopharyngeal myotomy which is adequate treatment for small diverticula. For large diverticula, myotomy with suspension or excision of the diverticulum is indicated (Fig. 6.3). Both these procedures provide similar good outcome in more than 90% of patients with a low incidence of complications. Simple excision of the diverticulum

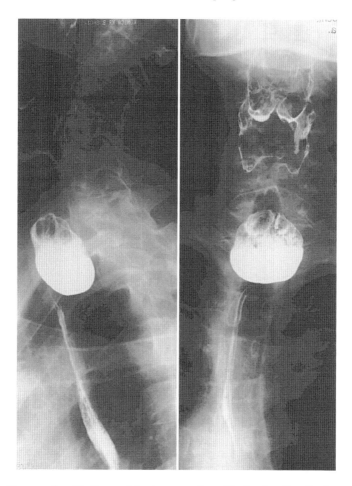

FIGURE 6.2. Radiographic image of a Zenker's diverticulum (Modified from Stein et al., 2006. With permission of Springer Science and Business Media).

without myotomy will result in c. diverticulectomy; d. status after myotomy and diverticulectomy; e. status after myotomy and pexy of the diverticulum to the prevertebral fascia (Modified from Stein et al., 2006. With permission of Springer Science and Business Media) high leakage rates from the diverticulectomy site; on long-term follow up, recurrences of

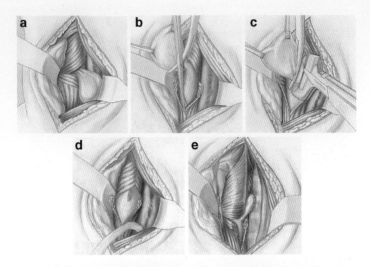

FIGURE 6.3. Classic open surgical approach to Zenker's diverticulum.
(**a**) Access and exposure; (**b**) cricopharyngeal myotomy; (**c**) excision
of diverticulum; (**d**) operative field after excision; (**e**) closure.

the diverticulum may occur, because the underlying pathogenetic mechanism has not been addressed.

More recently, minimally invasive, transoral endoscopic
methods have been described and are used increasingly. These
endoscopic techniques include transoral, endoscopic esophago-
diverticulostomy using a surgical stapler (Fig. 6.4) and transoral
division of the bridge between the esophagus and the diverticulum with a diathermic knife, laser, or argon plasma coagulation.

Despite some enthusiastic results from small series employing these techniques, a critical comparison shows that open
techniques probably afford better long-term symptomatic
relief than endoscopic approaches, especially in patients with
small diverticula.

## Midesophageal Diverticula

These more unusual diverticula are located in the middle
third of the esophagus within 4–5 cm proximal or distal to the
level of the carina. Until the late twentieth century,

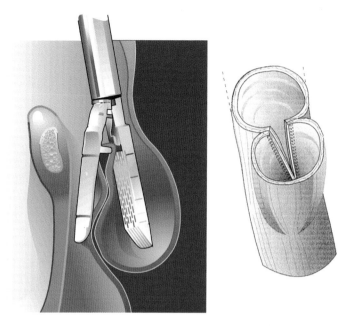

FIGURE 6.4. Schematic drawing of transoral stapling esophago-diverticulostomy for Zenker's diverticulum (Modified from Stein et al., 2006. With permission of Springer Science and Business Media).

midesophageal diverticula were caused commonly by traction due to mediastinal fibrosis or chronic lymphadenopathy from pulmonary tuberculosis or histoplasmosis. In the past, the majority of mid-esophageal diverticula were diagnosed incidentally in patients who had tuberculosis 20–30 years earlier. Because these diseases are far less common today and rarely progress to cause traction on the esophagus, patients presenting with a midesophageal diverticulum have become rare and, if no history of tuberculosis exists, should be evaluated for motility disorders of the esophageal body which may cause a pulsion diverticulum in this region.

Patients with midesophageal traction diverticula are usually asymptomatic; only the few with an excessively large diverticulum sack may report dysphagia, retrosternal pain, regurgitation, belching, epigastric pain, heartburn, and weight loss. In patients with a midesophageal pulsion diverticulum, symptoms may also result from an associated or underlying motor disorder or other underlying disease and not from the midthoracic diverticulum. Although complications are unusual, spontaneous rupture, iatrogenic perforation, exsanguination, aspiration, esophagobronchial fistula, and carcinoma have been reported.

Most patients with midesophageal diverticula require no treatment. Only in those with clear symptoms related to the diverticulum surgery is indicated. If no underlying motor disorder or esophageal obstruction is present, a simple resection of the diverticulum is the procedure of choice. Access through the right chest, via thoracotomy or thoracoscopy avoids the aortic arch and provides excellent exposure of the esophagus and airway at the tracheal bifurcation. Placing a bougie in the esophagus before excision of the diverticulum avoids compromise of the esophageal lumen. The diverticulum is resected with a stapling device. The closure may be buttressed with pleura, pleuropericardial fat pad, or omentum. An additional longitudinal myotomy of the esophagus distal to the origin of the diverticulum must be added in those with a pulsion diverticulum due to the underlying motor disorder (see below).

## Epiphrenic Diverticula

Epiphrenic diverticula are mucosal outpouchings of the esophageal wall that occur usually in the distal third of the esophagus. They are typically pulsion diverticula, that develop secondary to increased intraesophageal pressure, usually due to distal esophageal and/or lower esophageal sphincter motility disorders (such as achalasia, hypertensive lower esophageal sphincter or diffuse esophageal spasm).

The clinical manifestations of epiphrenic diverticula are variable with little correlation between the severity of symptoms and the size of the diverticulum. Distinguishing between symptoms of the diverticulum and those caused by the underlying motility disorder can be difficult.

A videotaped barium esophagogram best detects the presence of an epiphrenic diverticulum and often also allows characterization of the underlying motility disorder. Many patients show bizarre, non-propulsive tertiary contractions in the distal esophagus and/or a non-relaxing lower esophageal sphincter during the examination. In addition to the fixed, relatively wide-mouthed diverticulum, transient outpouchings can occur proximally in segments where peristalsis is absent. Endoscopy provides little information about diverticula but may be useful to assess associated esophageal problems like reflux disease. Manometry of the esophagus and the lower esophageal sphincter is mandatory to prove and classify the underlying motility disorder.

Only symptomatic epiphrenic diverticula are an indication for operation. Although good out-comes have been reported with diverticulectomy alone by some, the standard operation has become a distal esophageal myotomy (including the lower esophageal sphincter) in combination with a diverticulectomy. The myotomy will address the underlying motor disorder and avoid recurrences. Because myotomy across the lower esophageal sphincter is associated with a destruction of the physiologic antireflux mechanism, the addition of an antireflux procedure to diverticulectomy and myotomy is recommended. To avoid postoperative dysphagia, the added antireflux procedure should by only a partial fundoplication (e.g. a Dor or Toupet fundoplication). The classic approach is through the left chest, because this approach provides optimal access to the lower esophagus and esophagogastric junction. Recently, laparoscopic and thoracoscopic approaches to epiphrenic diverticula have been reported (Fig. 6.5). The complication rate of this approach in the few small published series is, however, relatively high, with fistula rates from the site of the diverticulectomy of up to 20%.

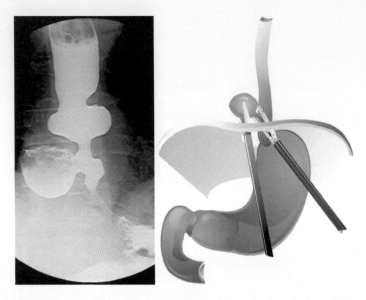

FIGURE 6.5.  Radiographic image of an epiphrenic diverticulum (left) and schematic drawing of a laparoscopic transhiatal approach for diverticulectomy (right) (Modified from Stein et al., 2006. With permission of Springer Science and Business Media).

## Selected Readings

Allen MS (1999) Treatment of epiphrenic diverticula. Semin Thorac Cardiovasc Surg 11:358–362

Bonavina L, Khan NA, DeMeester TR (1985) Pharyngoesophageal dysfunction: the role of cricopharyngeal myotomy. Arch Surg 120: 541–549

Fernando HC, Luketich JD, Samphire J et al. (2005) Minimally invasive operation for esophageal diverticula. Ann Thorac Surg 80: 2076–2081

Feussner H (2007) Endoscopic therapy for Zenker diverticulum - the good and the bad. Endoscopy 39:154–155

Gutschow CA, Hamoir M, Rombaux P et al. (2002) Management of pharyngoesophageal (Zenker's) diverticulum: which technique? Ann Thorac Surg 74:1677–1682

Nehra D, Lord RV, DeMeester TR et al. (2002) Physiologic basis for the treatment of epiphrenic diverticulum. Ann Surg 235:346–354

Omote K, Feussner H, Stein HJ, Siewert JR (1999) Endo-scopic stapling diverticulostomy for Zenker's diverticulum. Surg Endosc 13: 535–538

Rosati R, Fumagalli U, Bona S et al. (1998) Diverticulectomy, myotomy, and fundoplication through laparoscopy: a new option to treat epiphrenic esophageal diverticula? Ann Surg 227:174–178

Stein HJ, Feussner H, von Rahden BHA et al. (2006) Gutartige Erkrankungen von Ösophagus und Kardia. In: Siewert JR, Rothmund R, Schumpelick V (eds) Praxis der Viszerlachirurgie -Gastroenterologische Chirurgie, 2nd edn. Springer Medizin Verlag, Heidelberg, The Netherlands, pp. 241–294

Thomas ML, Anthony AA, Fosh BG et al. (2001) Oesophageal diverticula. Br J Surg 88:629–642

# Part II
# Esophagus and Paraesophageal Region: Malignant

# 7
# Esophageal Cancer: Diagnosis and Staging

**J. Rüdiger Siewert and Marcus Feith**

## Pearls and Pitfalls

- The aim of any diagnostic procedure is to identify the R0-resectable patient population.
- Topographic-anatomic localization and histologic proof of an esophageal cancer with endoscopy and biopsy is the essential diagnostic step.
- For squamous cell carcinoma of the esophagus, exclusion of a tracheo-bronchial fistula is required by esophageal contrast radiography, spiral computed tomography (CT), or bronchoscopy.
- Exclusion of distant metastases is best achieved with multislice spiral CT and/or positron emission tomography (PET).
- Diagnostic laparoscopy is the standard in advanced adenocarcinoma of the distal esophagus before embarking on multimodal approaches.
- The evaluation of the N-category before therapy remains a difficult and unreliable criteria for evaluation.
- T-category stage in esophageal cancer is best evaluated with endoscopic ultrasonography and is necessary for decision-making for further neoadjuvant, multimodal approaches.
- Synchronous carcinoma of the upper airways is common in squamous cell carcinoma and should be excluded by bronchoscopy and direct laryngoscopy.

K.I. Bland et al. (eds.), *Surgery of the Esophagus and Stomach*, DOI: 10.1007/978-1-84996-438-8_7,
© Springer-Verlag London Limited 2011

- Response prediction with a neoadjuvant therapeutic approach is essential to future therapeutic assessment.
- Quantitative measurements of tumor uptake by PET may allow the evaluation of the response to 2 weeks of neoadjuvant therapy.
- Preoperative risk analysis for patients with esophageal cancer defines factors essential to the planned therapeutic approach.
- With high global risk scores, a risk analysis of organ function related to the esophageal surgery is required.
- Patients with hepatic cirrhosis should be excluded generally from esophageal surgery.
- The composite risk score may be utilized to define the cardiorespiratory function and cervical and abdominal vascular status prior to the planned therapeutic protocol.

# Basic Diagnosis

As a consequence of dysphagia or other clinically relevant disorders of swallowing, the first diagnostic attempt is performed frequently by general practitioners or gastroenterologists. This is completed by primary endoscopy which leads directly to a diagnosis and histologic conformation. The x-ray or barium swallow is being used less often in recent years. The primary aim in diagnostic workup is to define the reasons for dysphagia. A more detailed diagnosis can be established subsequently. Thus, a comprehensive approach to diagnosis is necessary, because the questions which need to be answered differ widely. (Primary diagnosis: What is the reason for dysphagia? Secondary diagnosis: Is the tumor resectable? Is there evidence of distant metastases?)

Normally a biopsy is taken at the time of the first endoscopy. The discovery of a malignancy of the esophagus is the reason for sending the patient to the oncologist or surgeon. The best therapeutic approach is to refer the patient to an multidisciplinary center in a hospital with comprehensive experience in the treatment of esophageal malignancies ("High Volume Hospitals"). The secondary diagnostic staging can be performed in such a center and is then completed in a logical order.

## Specific Diagnosis

The aim of any diagnostic procedure with therapeutic relevance is to identify the R0-resectable patient population. The major operative aim is to achieve complete macroscopic and microscopic tumor resection (Table 7.1). These patients should be included in surgical therapeutic protocols. The following diagnostic information is necessary for an individualized decision formulation.

### First Step: Topographic-Anatomic Localization and Histology of the Primary Tumor

The first diagnostic step needed to achieve a specific diagnosis of esophageal carcinoma is a repeat endoscopy with multiple biopsies of the primary cancer. Chromoendoscopy with methylene blue and Lugol iodine will enhance the endoscopic determination of extent, thereby allowing directed biopsies of macroscopically nonvisible early carcinoma and will enhance the identification of sites of multicentric tumor growth. The biopsy is important for verification of histologic type, tumor differentiation, and subsequent tumor grading; this biopsy specimen may be used for future evaluation of molecular prognostic factors.

From the surgeon's perspective, the main criterion for resectability of squamous cell carcinoma of the esophagus is its anatomic relation to the tracheo-bronchial system. With growth, contact of the primary tumor with the tracheo-bronchial system or with evidence of a tracheo-bronchial fistula suggests that curative surgical resection is not possible. The combined resection of esophagus including parts of the tracheo-bronchial system or even a pneumonectomy is technically possible but prognostically ineffective. These advanced surgical approaches are obsolete in the paradigm of the

TABLE 7.1. Independent prognostic factors after resection of esophageal cancer (n = 1285). A multivariate analysis.

| | B | SE | Wald | df | Significance | Exp (B) |
|---|---|---|---|---|---|---|
| Adenocarcinoma/squamous cell carcinoma | 0.696 | 0.132 | 27.641 | 1 | 0 | 2.005 |
| Sex | −0.269 | 0.147 | 3.324 | 1 | 0.068 | 0.764 |
| Age | 0.011 | 0.045 | 4.374 | 1 | 0.036 | 1.011 |
| Lymph nodes positive | 0.036 | 0.007 | 24.07 | 1 | 0 | 1.037 |
| Lymph nodes total | −0.011 | 0.004 | 7.741 | 1 | 0.005 | 0.989 |
| pN (lymph nodes) | 0.573 | 0.102 | 31.791 | 1 | 0 | 1.773 |
| M (distant metastases) | 0.284 | 0.144 | 3.908 | 1 | 0.048 | 1.329 |
| R (residual tumor) | 0.56 | 0.094 | 35.817 | 1 | 0 | 1.752 |
| G (grading) | 0.071 | 0.078 | 0.824 | 1 | 0.364 | 1.073 |
| pT (tumor infiltration) | 0.309 | 0.06 | 26.39 | 1 | 0 | 1.863 |
| Postoperative complications | 0.569 | 0.101 | 34.747 | 1 | 0 | 1.814 |

present oncologic approach to esophageal surgery for esophageal cancer.

Especially problematic are esophageal tumors localized in direct relation to the trachea. The tissue layer between esophagus and trachea is very thin; a complete R0-resection is only possible in early carcinoma (T1/T2 infiltration).

To identify the relation of esophageal carcinoma to the tracheo-bronchial system, use of high resolution, multislice spiral CT for study of the mediastinum is recommended. Also, esophageal contrast radiography identifies the relationship of the primary tumor to the tracheal bifurcation. The contrast radiogram will provide evidence optimally of an existing fistula of the tracheo-bronchial system to the mediastinum. Endoscopic ultrasonography (EUS) is ineffective for the diagnosis of tracheo-bronchial infiltration of esophageal carcinoma because of the reduced ability to visualize the airway system.

## Second Step: Exclusion of Distant Metastases

In the presence of distant metastases, a surgical resection, even with palliative intent, is unreasonable. In practice, the authors exclude the presence of liver and pulmonary metastases by CT. The fluorodeoxyglucose-positron emission tomography (FDG-PET) is used increasingly to evaluate for distant tumor spread. The FDG-PET is utilized currently for assessment of therapeutic response for prediction of patient outcome after neoadjuvant therapy; therefore, a pretherapeutic FDG-PET is required.

In our opinion, skeletal scintigraphy (bone scan) is not useful in the primary diagnostic approach. Similarly, a bone marrow biopsy to identify isolated tumor cells is only practicable for use in randomized experimental therapeutic studies.

Use of diagnostic laparoscopy in patients with squamous cell carcinoma of the esophagus is of value only to exclude hepatic cirrhosis. In contrast, 30% of patients with adenocarcinoma of the distal esophagus are confirmed with diagnostic laparoscopy to harbor occult liver metastases or the presence of peritoneal carcinomatosis despite the false-negative staging information that results with CT (Table 7.2). Diagnostic

TABLE 7.2. Information in diagnostic laparoscopy in squamous cell carcinoma or adenocarcinoma of the esophagus (Stein et al., 1997).

| | Liver metastases | Peritoneal carcinosis | Tumor cells in abdominal lavage | Liver cirrhosis |
|---|---|---|---|---|
| Squamous cell carcinoma of the esophagus | | | | |
| T1/T2-tumor | 0/19 (0%) | 0/19 (0%) | 0/19 (0%) | 2/19 (11%) |
| T3/T4-tumor | 3/36 (8%) | 0/36 (0%) | 0/36 (0%) | 5/36 (14%) |
| Adenocarcinoma of the distal esophagus | | | | |
| T1/T2-tumor | 1/9 (11%) | 0/9 (0%) | 0/9 (0%) | 0/9 (0%) |
| T3/T4-tumor | 4/16 (25%) | 3/16 (19%) | 4/16 (25%) | 0/16 (0%) |

laparoscopy, thus, remains the standard staging approach for advanced adenocarcinoma of the distal esophagus, i.e. before a multimodal approach.

## Third Step (Staging In Detail): T-and N-Category of the Primary Tumor

After exclusion of distant metastases in esophageal carcinoma, the therapeutic approach is influenced by the T-category (Table 7.3). The evaluation of the N-category preoperatively is difficult, and data obtained radiographically may be unreliable. Thus, prediction of tumor infiltration in lymph nodes is based principally on the size of the lymph nodes. Direct biopsy of lymph nodes via medianoscopy, thoracotomy, or CT is ill-advised, because regional lymph node metastases do not represent a contraindication for surgery.

The "gold standard" to evaluate the T-category in esophageal carcinoma is the EUS. The predictive value of the T-category with EUS by experienced examiners exceeds 80%. The presence of stenosis secondary to tumor

TABLE 7.3. Prevalence of lymph node metastases in adenocarcinoma or squamous cell carcinoma of the esophagus in relation to the pT-category (resected patients at the department of surgery of the Technical University Munich).

|  | Squamous cell carcinoma of the esophagus | Adenocarcinoma of the esophagus |
| --- | --- | --- |
| pT1-category |  |  |
| Mucosa pT1a | 8 | 0 |
| Submucosa pT1b | 36 | 20 |
| pT2-category | 58 | 67 |
| pT3-category | 74 | 85 |
| pT4-category | 79 | 89 |

TABLE 7.4. Diagnostic procedures in esophageal carcinoma.

| Diagnostic procedure | Question |
|---|---|
| Obligate diagnostic endoscopy and biopsy | Tumor growth and histology |
| Multislice spiral computed tomography/esophageal contrast radiogram | Localization and relation to tracheo-bronchial system |
| CT scan thorax and abdominal | Exclusion of distant metastases |
| Additional diagnostic procedures | |
| Endoscopic ultrasonography | Determination of the T-category |
| Tracheoscopy and biopsy | By esophageal carcinoma with direct localization to the tracheobronchial system: exclusion of infiltration |
| Diagnostic laparoscopy | By advanced (T3/T4) primary adenocarcinoma: exclusion of liver or peritoneal metastases |
| Direct laryngoscopy | In squamous cell carcinoma: exclusion of synchronous carcinoma of the upper airways |

infiltration is a indication of an advanced tumor stage (T3/T4). Additional information of the topographic anatomy, extraluminal growth characteristics, and relationship to surrounding organs is evident with EUS. Conclusions regarding the N-category and R0-resectability are possible via inference from the T-category. With the new multislice spiral CT, enhanced staging criteria for the T-category have been reported (Table 7.4).

## Special Diagnostic Aspects

- Exclusion of synchronous carcinoma of the upper airway in esophageal carcinoma.

Synchronous carcinoma of the upper airways is evident in as many as 10% of patients with squamous cell carcinoma of the esophagus. To exclude synchronous carcinoma, we suggest a bronchoscopy and direct laryngoscopy.

- Response prediction and response evaluation in neoadjuvant therapeutic approaches.

Because only patients with an objective response to neoadjuvant chemotherapy or combination radiochemotherapy benefit from multimodal therapeutic approaches, response prediction remains a subject of active investigation. Actually, only tumor grading represents a clear "predictor" for the outcome after neoadjuvant therapy. Importantly, the presence of the G4-grading or of small cell tumor components in the pretherapeutic biopsy enhances the success of chemotherapy. In studies, the level of ERCC-1-gene expression and thymidylate-synthase activity of the tumor showed remarkable results for the evaluation of response to neoadjuvant polychemotherapy. Unfortunately, definitive, reliable parameters do not exist for the prediction of clinical response or that expected in conventional imaging for patients after use of neoadjuvant chemotherapy or irradiation treatment.

Thus, the identification of novel parameters that predict response and prognosis are crucial for future therapeutic interventions. Post-therapeutic assessment of tumor response by FDG-PET has been shown to correlate with histopathologic tumor regression and patient survival. Furthermore, quantitative measurements of tumor FDG-uptake may allow an early evaluation of the metabolic response to neoadjuvant therapy after only 2 weeks of therapy.

## Risk Analysis

Major risk assessment for patients with esophageal carcinoma must include preservation of organ function related to the

TABLE 7.5. Selection of the therapeutic approach based on pretherapeutic assessment of the resectability of the tumor and functional analysis.

| General condition | RO-resection possible | RO-resection questionable | Infiltration tracheo-bronchial and/or distant metastases |
|---|---|---|---|
| Good | Primary resection | Multimodal therapy | Palliation |
| Compromised | Primary resection | Multimodal therapy or definitive CTx/RCTx | Palliation |
| Severely impaired | Definitive CTx/RCTx Local access (stent, laser therapy) | Definitive CTx/RCTx Local access (stent, laser therapy) | Palliation |

esophageal surgery (Table 7.5). Global risk scores reported in the literature fail principally to evaluate operative risk. In squamous cell carcinoma of the esophagus, preoperative risk analysis includes factors that influence therapeutic decisions. The epidemiologic correlate of a high incidence of alcohol abuse in patients with squamous cell carcinoma of the esophagus requires the analysis of liver function; the exclusion of more advanced cirrhosis (Childs B or C), with all diagnostic approaches (serum albumin, coagulation tests, aminopyrine breath test) and morphologic examination (ultrasonography, CT), including liver biopsy, may be required. Biochemical, radiologic, and histologic evidence of cirrhosis is a relative contraindication to surgical resection of esophageal carcinoma.

Respiratory function has to be evaluated prior to resection of esophageal carcinoma; however, these results provide only a marginal influence on the surgical approach, because postoperative use of respiratory therapy is routine. A detailed evaluation of cardiac and vascular function is recommended in any patient considered for esophagectomy in whom the

TABLE 7.6. Composite risk score system (Bartels, 1998).

| Parameters | Preoperative classification[a] | Weighting factor | Minimum score | Maximum score |
|---|---|---|---|---|
| General status | 1/2/2003 | 4 | 4 | 12 |
| Cardiac function | 1/2/2003 | 3 | 3 | 9 |
| Liver function | 1/2/2003 | 2 | 2 | 6 |
| Pulmonary function | 1/2/2003 | 2 | 2 | 6 |
| Composite score | | | 11 | 33 |

[a]Preoperative classification: 1 normal, 2 compromised, 3 severely impaired.

history, physical examination, chest radiograph, or standard electrocardiogram show any abnormality.

Establishment of a useful risk analysis especially for patients with squamous cell carcinoma of the esophagus categorizes objectively the general status, compliance, and cooperation of the individual patient for these extended surgical procedures. It is imperative to establish the presence preoperatively of chronic alcohol abuse at the time of surgery; the postoperative morbidity is as great as 50% in chronic alcohol abuse. The diagnosis of alcoholism within standard clinical routine may be difficult; in most cases, the treatment of alcohol-related diseases and complications is protracted.

In summary, the risk of esophagectomy in patients with potentially resectable esophageal cancer can be assessed objectively before operative treatment and quantified by the composite risk score (Table 7.6). Strict inclusion of the risk score in the preoperative decision-making process decreases the postoperative morbidity and mortality. Patients should only be referred for esophagectomy if the risk score reflects a relatively healthy and cooperative patient. In our own experience, up to 30% of the patient population is excluded because of a negative preoperative composite risk score (Figs. 7.1 and 7.2).

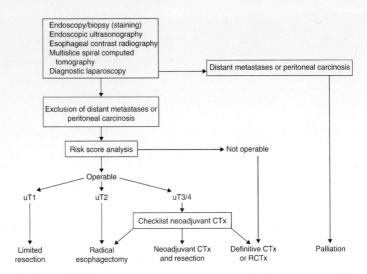

FIGURE 7.1. Diagnostic flow sheet adenocarcinoma (Barrett carcinoma) of the distal esophagus.

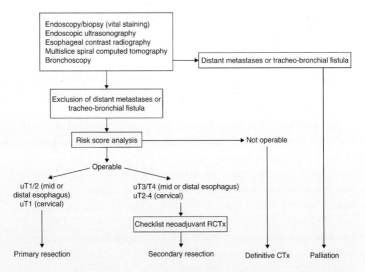

FIGURE 7.2. Diagnostic flow sheet squamous cell carcinoma of the esophagus.

# Selected Readings

Bartels H, Stein HJ, Siewert JR (1998) Preoperative risk analysis and postoperative mortality of oesophagectomy for resectable oesophageal cancer. Br J Surg 85:840–844

Dittler HJ, Siewert JR (1993) Role of endoscopic ultrasonography in esophageal carcinoma. Endoscopy 25:156–161

Feith M, Stein HJ, Siewert JR (2006) Adenocarcinoma of the esophagogastric junction: surgical therapy based on 1602 consecutive resected patients. Surg Oncol Clin N Am 15:751–764

Ott K, Weber W, Siewert JR (2006) The importance of PET in the diagnosis and response evaluation of esophageal cancer. Dis Esophagus. 19:433–442

Riedel M, Hauck RW, Stein HJ et al. (1998) Preoperative bronchoscopic assessment of airway invasion by esophageal cancer: a prospective study. Chest. 113(3):687–695

Siewert JR, Stein HJ, Feith M et al. (2001) Histologic tumor type is an independent prognostic parameter in esophageal cancer: lessons from more than 1000 consecutive resections at a Single Center in the Western World. Ann Surg 234:360–369

Siewert JR, Stein HJ, Feith M (2003) Surgical approach to invasive adenocarcinoma of the distal esophagus (Barrett's cancer). World J Surg 27:1058–1061

Stein HJ, Feith M (2001) Prognostic factors in cancer of the esophagus. In: Gospodarowicz MK, Henson DE, Hutter RVP et al. (eds) Prognostic factors in cancer. Wiley-Liss, New York, pp. 237–249

Stein HJ, Kraemer SJ, Feussner H et al. (1997) Clinical value of diagnostic laparoscopy with laparoscopic ultrasound in patients with cancer of the esophagus or cardia. J Gastrointest Surg 1:167–172

# 8
# Esophageal Cancer: Transhiatal Resection

**Hubert J. Stein**

## Pearls and Pitfalls

- A wide-splitting of the esophageal hiatus and use of special retractors allows good access to the distal esophagus and lower posterior mediastinum.
- Radical resection of the distal esophagus and lymphadenectomy of the lower posterior mediastinum can be achieved transhiatally up to the level of the tracheal bifurcation.
- Transhiatal, distal esophageal resection and transhiatal, subtotal esophageal resection are safer than thoracoabdominal approaches.
- For most patients with adenocarcinoma of the distal esophagus or esophagogastric junction, transhiatal resection has equivalent outcomes to transthoracic approaches.
- The use of circular stapling devices allows safe construction of esophageal anastomoses through the esophageal hiatus after transhiatal distal esophageal resection.
- The cervical anastomosis remains the "Achilles' heel" of transhiatal subtotal esophagectomy.
- In patients with early esophageal cancer *without* lymph node metastases, a transhiatal resection with preservation of the vagus and undiseased esophagus should be considered as the standard of care.

K.I. Bland et al. (eds.), *Surgery of the Esophagus and Stomach*, DOI: 10.1007/978-1-84996-438-8_8,
© Springer-Verlag London Limited 2011

# Introduction

Numerous approaches exist for removing the esophagus in patients with esophageal cancer, most requiring access through the left or right chest in addition to alaparotomy. Removal of the intrathoracic esophagus in a patient with esophageal cancer without thoracotomy by employing a transabdominal/transhiatal and transcervical approach was first performed successfully by the British surgeon Turner in the 1930s at a time when thoracotomy was associated with a formidable mortality risk. After the introduction of endotracheal anesthesia and safe techniques of thoractomy, which permitted transthoracic esophagectomy under direct vision, the technique of transhiatal esophagectomy was almost abandoned for years and used only for removal of a "healthy esophagus" in patients with cervical esophageal cancer, for palliation of incurable esophageal cancer, and for patients with caustic, pharyngo-esophageal strictures. In the 1980s, esophagectomy without thoracotomy was "rediscovered" and perfected and popularized subsequently by Orringer et al. as a safer alternative to abdomino-thoracic or thoracoabdominal approaches for cancer at virtually every level of the esophagogastric junction and the esophagus. Because the focus of Orringer's approach was clearly to minimize the morbidity of esophagectomy and to palliate malignant dysphagia, others claimed that this approach "ignored" some of the classic principles of cancer surgery (i.e. wide local excision and lymphadenectomy), and therefore the role of transhiatal resection of esophageal cancer as a curative procedure remained controversial.

Clear local resection margins and lymph node status are the dominant prognostic factors after surgical resection in patients with esophageal cancer. The prevalence and patterns of lymphatic spread of esophageal cancer have been shown to be related closely to the depth of invasion, histologic tumor type, and location of the primary neoplasm in the esophagus. Because systematic lymphadenectomy in the upper abdomen and lower posterior mediastinum, but not in the upper mediastinum, is possible with a transhiatal resection, a more differentiated view of the role of the various resection techniques and surgical approaches has emerged recently.

Tumor biology, pattern of lymphatic spread, type of affected patients, and prognosis after surgical resection differs markedly between adenocarcinoma of the esophagogastric junction, adenocarcinoma of the distal esophagus, and squamous cell cancer of the thoracic esophagus. Surgical strategies for treatment of adenocarcinoma arising in the distal esophagus or the vicinity of the esophagogastric junction, therefore, must be planned differently from those for squamous cell cancer of the intrathoracic esophagus. In particular, a subtotal esophagectomy is rarely necessary to achieve a clear proximal margin for a distal esophageal adenocarcinoma or adenocarcinoma of the esophagogastric junction invading the distal esophagus. These concepts are in marked contrast to those in squamous cell esophageal cancer, where extensive submucosal spread and multicentricity within the entire esophagus is not uncommon. Furthermore, in contrast to squamous cell esophageal cancer, lymphatic metastases are found predominantly in the lower posterior mediastinum and upper abdomen in patients with adenocarcinoma of the distal esophagus or esophagogastric junction. While at most centers a transthoracic approach with subtotal esophagectomy and systematic mediastinal lymphadenectomy is considered standard for patients with squamous cell esophageal cancer, a distal esophageal resection with lymphadenectomy of the lower posterior mediastinum and upper abdomen may suffice for many, if not most, patients with adenocarcinoma at or close to the esophagogastric junction.

Based on these data, the surgical approaches to esophageal cancer should be tailored to the required oncologic radicality for complete tumor removal and locoregional lymph node clearance. The perceived benefits of surgical radicality must then be balanced against the risk of the procedure. With this concept, transhiatal approaches to the esophagus have a firm place in the armamentarium of individualized surgical treatment strategies for esophageal cancer, particularly in patients with adenocarcinoma of the distal esophagus or esophagogastric junction.

Three entirely different approaches are referred to as "transhiatal esophageal resection" or "esophageal resection without thoracotomy":

1. Transhiatal resection of the distal esophagus with an anastomosis to the remnant esophagus performed transhiatally in the lower posterior mediastinum
2. Transhiatal subtotal esophagectomy with an anastomosis to the remnant cervical esophagus performed in the neck
3. Limited and vagal-sparing transhiatal esophageal resection for early carcinoma without lymph node metastases

These procedures differ markedly in the extent of esophageal resection and lymphadenectomy and must be differentiated when discussing the merits and risks of "transhiatal resection."

## Transhiatal Resection of the Distal Esophagus with Lower Mediastinal Anastomosis

In patients with adenocarcinoma at or in the vicinity of the esophagogastric junction, a subtotal esophagectomy is required only rarely to achieve clear proximal resection margins. Rather, a complete resection of the primary tumor can in most instances also be achieved with clear proximal margins via a transhiatal access through a laparotomy only. Furthermore, lymphatic spread of such neoplasms is directed predominantly toward the lower posterior mediastinum and the upper abdomen. Consequently, in most instances, there is no need to perform a lymphadenectomy of the proximal mediastinum. A wide anterior or left lateral splitting of the esophageal hiatus and insertion of specially designed, extra-long retractors through the hiatus into the mediastinum allows good access up to the level of the tracheal bifurcation and facilitates complete clearance of the lymphatic tissue in the lower posterior mediastinum

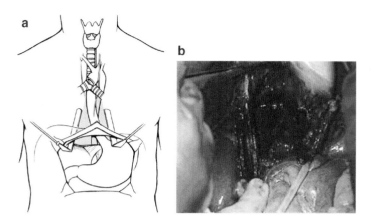

FIGURE 8.1. Wide exposure of the distal esophagus and lower posterior mediastinum after splitting of the esophageal hiatus. (**a**) graphic depiction. (**b**) intraoperative view. (**a** figure modified from Siewert et al., 2006. With kind permission of Springer Science and Business Media).

(Fig. 8.1). Resection of upto 10 cm of the distal esophagus together with a lymphadenectomy up to the tracheal bifurcation is possible through this approach. Circular stapler devices allow a safe anastomosis with the remnant esophagus in the lower mediastinum without thoracotomy (Fig. 8.2).

In the author's experience, the oncologic results and the long-term outcome of this approach are at least as good as those with the more radical abdomino-thoracic procedures with a two-field or three-field lymphadenectomy, while the surgical procedure was safer and the postoperative course smoother when thoracotomy was avoided. This experience was recently confirmed by a prospective, randomized study from the National Cancer Center in Tokyo. In this study, the abdominothoracic approach was associated with a higher postoperative mortality rate and a significantly higher postoperative overall morbidity as compared to the transhiatal approach. There were no significant differences in long-term survival between the two procedures. Thus, a thoracotomy with subtotal esophagectomy and proximal mediastinal

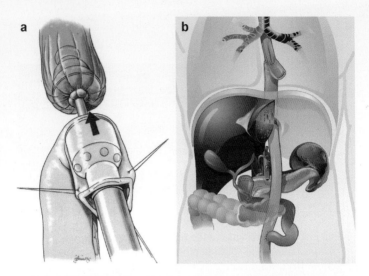

FIGURE 8.2. Esophago-intestinal end-to-side anastomosis in the lower posterior mediastinum after transhiatal distal esophageal resection. (**a**) end-to-side anastomosis with a circular stapler device. (**b**) graphic depiction of a completed esophagojejunostomy immediately below the level of the tracheal bifurcation after total gastrectomy and trans-hiatal resection of the distal esophagus.

lymphadenectomy is not necessary for the vast majority of patients with adenocarcinoma of the gastric cardia or subcardiac region, even when distal esophageal invasion is present. The thoracotomy only adds morbidity without a survival benefit. Rather, a pure transabdominal/transhiatal approach is the access of choice, whenever a clear oral resection margin can be achieved by this procedure.

# Transhiatal Subtotal Esophagectomy with Cervical Anastomosis

Transhiatal subtotal esophagectomy with a cervical anastomosis is the procedure popularized by Orringer and colleagues in the early 1980s. Although the principles of surgical oncology for procedures aiming at cure (wide local excision and lymph-adenectomy) argue against the use of this procedure for patients with intrathoracic squamous cell cancer, the advantage of this approach for patients with adenocarcinoma of the distal esophagus which cannot be resected completely through an abdominal approach alone. Additionally, another indication for the approach is evident with poor pulmonary function who may not tolerate thoracotomy. The procedure encompasses both an abdominal and transhiatal mobilization and cervical esophago-gastric anastomosis. In modification of Orringer's more palliative viewpoint, a wide splitting of the esophageal hiatus and retraction of the diaphragmatic crura laterally and the heart anteriorly also allows a lymphadenectomy of the lower posterior mediastinum and wide local excision of distal esophageal neoplasms. "Enbloc" mobilization of the distal esophagus and all surrounding tissues including both mediastinal pleural sheets is possible under direct vision up to the level of the tracheal bifurcation (Fig. 8.3). The "blind" and "blunt" phase of the operation is then restricted to only a few centimeters of the retrotracheal, intrathoracic esophagus

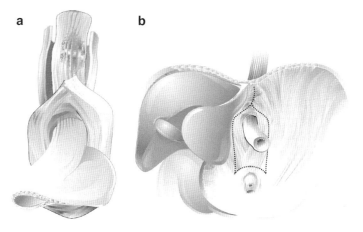

FIGURE 8.3. Wide local excision (**a**) of the  distal esophagus and stomach with (**b**) transhiatal approach and excision of hiatal part of the diaphragm.

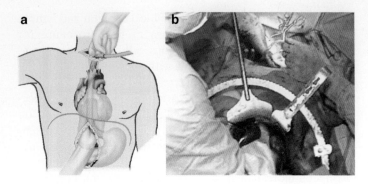

FIGURE 8.4. The "blunt" and "blind" phase of transhiatal subtotal esophagectomy via an abdominal and cervical incision. (**a**) graphic depiction. (**b**) intraoperative view: two fingers of the left hand of the surgeon mobilize the proximal intrathoracic esophagus from the posterior wall of the trachea. The right hand is inserted into the mediastinum through the hiatus mobilizing the proximal esophagus from below (**a** figure modified from Siewert et al., 2006. With kind permission of Springer Science and Business Media).

(Fig. 8.4). With the use of a modified mediastinoscope inserted through the neck incision, this part of the operation may also be performed under controlled conditions and lymph node biopsies in this area becomes possible. Nevertheless, even with this technical support, one must realize that a formal lymph-adenectomy in the upper mediastinum will not possible with the transhiatal and transcervical access.

The need for a cervical anastomosis remains the major problem of this procedure. Although cervical anastomotic leaks pose a lesser problem during the postoperative course compared with intrathoracic anastomotic leaks, cervical leaks are more common and usually result in strictures requiring repeated dilatations.

Recently, a large, prospective, randomized trial from the Netherlands by Hulscher and colleagues compared transhiatal subtotal esophagectomy with abdominothoracic esophagectomy in patients with adenocarcinoma of the distal esophagus or gastric cardia. Transhiatal subtotal esophagectomy was associated with fewer postoperative complications (in particular pulmonary complications), shorter postoperative mechanical ventilation time, a shorter postoperative stay in an intensive care unit, and a shorter overall hospital stay. Although survival analysis showed a trend toward a prognostic benefit in the patients with a more radical abdominothoracic approach, this difference was not significant on statistical analysis. Compared with abdominothoracic esophagectomy, a transhiatal subtotal esophagectomy has been established to be a less invasive and a safer approach to patients with adenocarcinoma of the distal esophagus orgastric cardia, without a significant loss in long-term prognosis. This technique, therefore, can be advocated for patients with distal esophageal adenocarcinoma particularly if, due to preexisting comorbidity, a thoracotomy is perceived as hazardous or risky, and a transhiatal resection of the distal esophagus alone does not permit complete tumor removal.

# Limited and Vagal-Sparing Transhiatal Esophageal Resection for Early Esophageal Carcinoma without Lymph Node Metastases

Due to endoscopic surveillance programs and an increased awareness in industrialized nations, esophageal cancer is diagnosed increasingly at early stages, particularly in patients with known precancerous lesions, e.g. Barrett's esophagus. Large studies indicate that lymph node metastases are virtually absent if the neoplasm is limited to the mucosa. Consequently, systematic lymphadenectomy is not needed in such patients. Many of these patients are treated by endoscopic ablation or endoscopic resection. These endoscopic techniques, however, do not address the underlying precancerous epithelium or the multicentricity of such neoplasms. Recurrences are common after endoscopic intervention for early esophageal cancer. Because no lymphatic spread is anticipated in such patients, more limited, local techniques of resection with lesser morbidity preserve more healthy esophagus and minimize organ dysfunction and are thus suited

ideally for these patients. Transhiatal approaches to esophageal resection meet these requirements. Several such procedures have been reported in recent years. In patients with
early adenocarcinoma or a high grade intraepithelial neopla-
sia ("high grade dysplasia") arising in Barrett's esophagus, a
limited transhiatal resection of the distal esophageal segment
affected with the Barrett's metaplasia and reconstruction
with jejunal interposition provides cure and preserves undiseased esophagus (Fig. 8.5). Because vagal innervation of the
upper gastrointestinal tract and the gastric reservoir function
can be preserved, this approach is associated with a very good

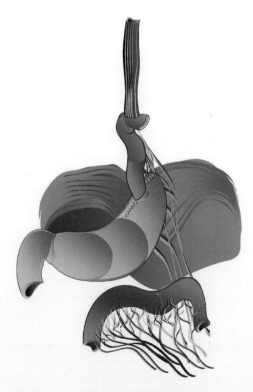

FIGURE 8.5. Graphic depiction of a limited transhiatal distal esophageal resection with jejunal interposition.

quality of life. Vagal-sparing, subtotal transhiatal esophagectomy is another alternative in such patients with a reported very good quality of life.

## Summary

Transhiatal approaches to esophageal resection have been proven to be safer than abdominothoracic esophagectomy. In patients with adenocarcinoma of the distal esophagus and esophagogastric junction, a transhiatal resection of the distal esophagus in combination with lymphadenectomy of the lower posterior mediastinum is oncologically equivalent to more radical procedures employing thoracotomy and systematic mediastinal lymph node dissection. With modern circular stapling devices, safe anastomoses with the esophageal remnant can be performed transhiatally up to the level of the tracheal bifurcation. The cervical anastomosis remains the "Achilles' heel" of transhiatal subtotal esophagectomy. In patients with early esophageal cancer without lymphatic spread, transhiatal vagal-sparing approaches should be the standard of care.

## Selected Readings

Banki F, Mason RJ, DeMeester SR et al. (2002) Vagal-sparing esophagectomy: a more physiologic alternative. Ann Surg 236:324–336

Bumm R, Feussner H, Bartels H et al. (1997) Radical trans-hiatal esophagectomy with two-field lymphadenectomy and endodissection for distal esophageal adenocarcinoma. World J Surg 21:822–831

Hulscher JB, van Sandick JW, de Boer AG et al. (2002) Extended transthoracic resection compared with limited transhiatal resection for adenocarcinoma of the esophagus. N Engl J Med 347:1662–1669

Kitajima M, Kitagawa Y (2002) Surgical treatment of esophageal cancer - the advent of the era of individualization. N Engl J Med 347:1705–1709

Orringer MB, Marshall B, Iannettoni MD (1999) Transhiatal esophagectomy: clinical experience and refinements. Ann Surg 230:392–404

Sasako M, Sano T, Yamamoto S et al. (2006) Left thoracoabdominal approach versus abdominal transhiatal approach for gastric cancer of the cardia or subcardia: a randomised controlled trial. Lancet Oncol 7:644–651

Siewert JR, Feith M, Werner M, Stein HJ (2000) Adenocarcinoma of the esophagogastric junction. Results of surgical therapy based on anatomical/topographic classification in 1,002 consecutive patients. Ann Surg 232:353–361

Siewert JR, Stein HJ, Feith M (2006) Ösophaguskarzinom. In: Siewert JR, Rothmun M, Schumpelick V (eds) Praxis der Viszeralchirurgie, Siewert Onkologische Chirurgie, 2nd edn. Springer-Verlag, Heidelberg, pp 403–434

Stein HJ, Feith M, Brücher BLDM et al. (2005) Early esophageal cancer: pattern of lymphatic spread and prognostic factors for long term survival after surgical resection. Ann Surg 242:566–572

# 9
# Transthoracic Esophagectomy

**Toni Lerut, Willy Coosemans, Georges Decker,
Paul De Leyn, Philippe Nafteux, and Dirk Van Raemdonck**

## Pearls and Pitfalls

- Lymphatic dissemination occurs early in the natural history of cancer of the esophagus and gastroesophageal junction.
- The pattern of lymphatic dissemination is difficult to predict, irrespective of the localization of the primary tumor.
- Intramural "jump-metastases" are common because of an extensive submucosal lymphatic plexus.
- Wide periesophageal "en bloc" resection and extensive two-field lymphadenectomy (three-field lymphadenectomy for middle-and proximal-third carcinomas) offer superior technique to obtain a macroscopic and microscopic complete R0 resection.
- Because of the preferential cephalad lymphatic dissemination, right-sided transthoracic esopha-gectomy is the preferred approach for supracarinal tumors.
- Distal-third esophageal and gastroesophageal junction cancers often have lymphatic dissemination along the lesser curvature toward the celiac axis. The left thoracoabdominal approach provides excellent exposure to combine radical resection in the chest with a DII lymphadenectomy in the superior abdominal compartment.

K.I. Bland et al. (eds.), *Surgery of the Esophagus and Stomach*, DOI: 10.1007/978-1-84996-438-8_9,
© Springer-Verlag London Limited 2011

- Primary radical esophagectomy results in overall 5-year survival of 30–40% and 20–25% for advanced stage III and IV disease, respectively. These figures are the gold standard to which all other therapeutic modalities should be compared.
- One year following esophagectomy, quality of life scores return to baseline for the majority of patients.
- Minimally invasive thoracoscopic and laparoscopic esophagectomy may evolve to the preferred approach for early (T1) carcinoma of the esophagus and GE junction.

# Introduction

The surgical treatment strategy of esophageal carcinoma is complex and the long term outcome of surgical therapy is often disappointing. Surgical resection can be impeded by the contiguous anatomic relations of the esophagus with the trachea, both main-stem bronchi and, more distally, the pericardium, aorta, and diaphragm. A malignancy arising from the esophagus may easily invade these adjacent organs, which makes the tumor surgically unresectable. Additionally, lymphatic dissemination is an early event and has a negative influence on survival. Lymph node metastases are found in less than 5% of intramucosal tumors, but in 30–40% of submucosal tumors. The esophageal wall is characterized by an extensive submucosal lymphatic plexus, which supplies a drainage route for early dissemination and gives rise to "jump-metastases" (i.e. lymph nodes adjacent to the primary tumor are unaffected, but more distant-located lymph nodes contain metastases).

Transmural tumors are showing lymph node involvement in over 80% and the number of involved nodes increases with the volume of the tumor.

# Principles of Surgical Treatment

It is generally accepted that surgical resection should only be performed with curative intent. Resection is ill-advised when macroscopically incomplete, due to invasion of adjacent structures and/or non-resectable metastases are to be expected. Absolute contra-indications for esophagectomy include local tumor invasion of non-resectable neighboring structures (T4), carcinomatosis peritonei, hematogenous parenchymatous metastases involving the liver and non-resectable metastatic lymph nodes.

The pattern of lymphatic dissemination is difficult to predict, but carcinomas of the proximal and middle thirds of the esophagus preferably metastasize to the cervical region, whereas more distal-lying tumors and tumors of the gastro-esophageal junction more commonly metastasize to the lymph nodes around the celiac axis.

*Resectable metastatic lymph nodes* in the region of the primary tumor, including the celiac trunk and its trifurcation removed with distal third tumors and cervical nodes for middle and proximal tumors, are not necessarily a contra-indication for surgery. The presence of lymph node metastases, however, has a negative influence on survival, even following extensive lymphadenectomy.

Macroscopic as well as microscopic completeness (R0) of resection is the ultimate goal of esophagectomy. Thus, optimal pre-operative staging is of paramount importance as well as individual case presentation and discussion at the multidisciplinary tumor board.

Optimal staging today includes endoscopy and biopsy, which are followed with echoendoscopy, high resolution CT scan, and PET scan.

Before embarking on major surgery, careful evaluation of medical operability is essential. Indeed many patients present with a history of alcohol and tobacco abuse requiring careful evaluation of cardiovascular, pulmonary, and liver functions.

Early-stage lymphatic dissemination, as well as completeness of tumoral resection (R0), pose challenges for radical surgical treatment and are still debatable. The concept of extensive en bloc resections was reported in 1963 by Logan, but its associated mortality of more than 20% in the original report, discouraged general acceptance. Skinner and Akiyama reintroduced the concept of en bloc resection combined with extensive lymphadenectomy. Ultimately, they were able to reduce operative mortality to 5%, with 5-year survival rates of 18% and 42%, respectively.

*The radical en bloc resection*, as opposed to the *standard resection*, aims at performing the wide, radical peritumoral nodal resection of the middle and distal thirds of the posterior mediastinum.

*The two-field lymph node dissection.* The early lymphatic dissemination, by means of longitudinal spread along the esophagus via the submucosal plexus to the upper mediastinum and abdomen, has advanced the advocacy of Japanese researchers for the two-field lymphadenectomy. This approach provides wide local excision of the primary tumor with lymphadenectomy of the entire posterior mediastinum; this technique includes resection of subcarinal nodes and nodes along the left recurrent nerve and the brachiocephalic trunk. Lymph nodes contiguous with the celiac trunk, common hepatic and splenic arteries, as well as the lymph nodes along the lesser gastric curvature and lesser omentum, are included.

*The three-field lymph node dissection.* The pattern of lymphatic dissemination is not restricted to the thorax and abdomen. About 20% of the patients with distal tumors present with metastasis in the cervical region. This metastatic pattern initiated consideration of the three-field lymph node dissection. In this operation, besides the already mentioned removal of thoracic and abdominal nodes, the cervical field is dissected, includes the paraesophageal, carotid vessel adenopathy, and supraclavicular nodes.

These considerations on radicality of resection and extent of lymphadenectomy are the rationale that justifies the *transthoracic approach* as opposed to the *transhiatal approach*. The rationale for the transhiatal esophagectomy is merely based on an effort to decrease perioperative morbidity and possibly postoperative mortality. Recent observations indicate that the results of radical esophagectomy are superior to those formerly quoted; contemporary results suggest overall 5-year survival figures that approach 40%.

# Technique

Esophageal tumors situated in the proximal and middle thirds of the intrathoracic esophagus are probably best approached via the right thoracic cavity. In contrast, distal tumors and tumors of the gastro-esophageal junction are best approached from the left side.

When the transthoracic approach is used, double lumen endotracheal intubation with intra-operative deflation of the lung at the operative side greatly facilitates the dissection in the posterior mediastinum.

The most commonly used transthoracic approaches are the Ivor Lewis (two hole) and McKeown (three hole) right thoracic approach and the left-sided approach through a left thoracophrenolaparotomy.

## *Ivor Lewis Procedure (Esophagectomy with Dorsolateral Thoracotomy)*

The procedure can be started either by a laparotomy followed by thoracotomy or vice versa (Clark et al., 1994). When the operation is initiated by laparotomy, the procedure is commenced by mobilization of the stomach. The esophagus is mobilized in the hiatus. After resection of the lesser curvature, a gastric tube is fashioned. The abdominal part is completed with a lymphadenectomy of the superior abdominal compartment, i.e. the lymph nodes along the celiac trunk and its branches, the splenic and common hepatic artery (DII lymphadenectomy).

After closure of the laparotomy the patient is repositioned in the left lateral decubitus position and a standard posterolateral right thoracotomy is performed, entering the chest through the fifth intercostal space. This access allows a perfect visualization of the posterior mediastinum. The esophagus is removed en bloc with its adjacent structures and is dissected from the vertebral body to the pericardium

(Fig. 9.1). The resection includes the removal of all tumor bearing esophagus surrounded by a wide envelope of adjacent tissues. To do so, the azygos vein and its associated nodes are removed with the thoracic duct, subcarinal nodes, para-esophageal nodes, all in continuity with the resected esophagus. The resected specimen also incorporates the mediastinal pleura on both sides. When indicated for middle and proximal third carcinoma, a meticulous dissection of the lymph nodes along the left recurrent nerve and the brachiocephalic trunk may be performed in the same intervention. The gastric tube which has been temporarily fixed to the remainder of the lesser curvature is pulled into the chest; an

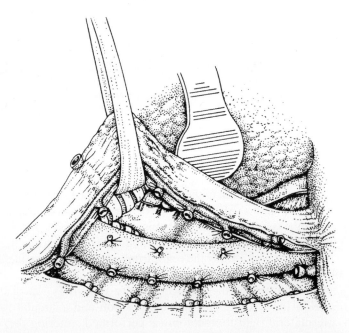

FIGURE 9.1. En bloc esophagectomy. All tissues surrounding the esophagus including azygos vein en thoracic duct are left on the specimen. The aorta shows its ligated intercostals vessels and esophageal bronchial arteries. The subcarinal nodes are removed en bloc with the specimen (Reprinted from Skinner, 1983. Copyright 1983. With permission from the American Association for Thoracic Surgery).

anastomosis is fashioned high in the apex of the chest will complete the procedure.

## McKeown Procedure (Esophagectomy with Anterolateral Thoracotomy and Cervical Anastomosis)

In this procedure the patient is placed in a supine position but with slight elevation of the right side of the chest (Hulscher et al., 2002; Fig. 9.2). This position allows for a synchronous

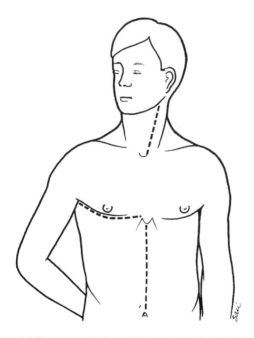

FIGURE 9.2. McKeown technique. Illustration of the incisions. The intervention can also be performed without having to turn the patient avoiding a need for repeat preparation and draping. The right thoracotomy is usually made in the fourth interspace (Reprinted from Pearson, 1995. Copyright 1995. With permission from Elsevier).

abdominal midline laparotomy. A right anterolateral thoracotomy in the fourth or fifth intercostal space and a cervical incision on either the right or left side. The technique of gastric mobilization, abdominal lymphadenectomy, and transthoracic mobilization of the esophagus is essentially the same as described in the previous operation. The anastomosis is performed via a separate left cervicotomy through which the proximal esophagus and the attached gastric tube are pulled up into the operative field. The main disadvantage of this operation is however that the extent of radicality; lymphadenectomy is more difficult to achieve as compared to the previously described technique.

## Left Thoracoabdominal Approach

The left thoracic approach is considered by many authors as the standard approach for carcinoma of the lower esophagus and cardia (Fig. 9.3). The operation was popularized by Sweet. The left postero-lateral approach may be extended anteriorly across the costal margin as advocated by Belsey. This provides a true thoracoabdominal exposure of both the superior abdominal compartment and posterior mediastinum. With this approach, the chest is entered through the sixth intercostal space. After dividing the costal margin, the diaphragm is incised at its periphery as an inverted T-shape incision, the short limb of the T incising the abdominal wall over a few centimeters. This approach allows an optimal direct vision for both the abdominal and chest cavities via one single incision. As a result, through this incision maximum exposure/resection can be achieved. The entire thoracic esophagus can be dissected through the left-sided approach. The dissection of the esophagus from beneath the aortic arch requires ligation and transection of the bronchial arteries just below the arch. The mobilization is then continued by blunt finger dissection behind the aortic arch and up into the apex of the chest. The mediastinal pleura above the aortic arch is opened. After transecting the esophagus at a level below the cardia, the esophagus is pulled and delivered through the

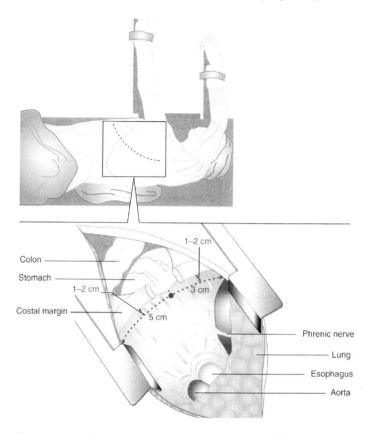

FIGURE 9.3. Left thoracoabdominal approach. The chest is entered through the sixth intercostal space. After dividing the costochondral margin an inverted T shaped incision is made in the diaphragm at its periphery taking care to avoid injury to the phrenic nerve (Reprinted from Lerut and Van Lanschot, 2004).

opened mediastinal pleura above the aortic arch and transected. Lymphadenectomy in both the abdomen and posterior mediastinum can be performed. After resecting the esophagus, the gastric tube is brought upward through the hiatus and behind the aortic arch and temporarily fixed to the esophageal stump in the apex of the chest. The incision is then closed and the patient is turned to a supine position. Through a left cervicotomy, the esophageal stump with the attached gastric tube is exteriorized into the operative field and a cervical esophagogastrostomy is performed. This cervical part of the operation can be combined with a bilateral lymphadenectomy (third field) through a U-shape incision in the neck. In the three-field lymphadenectomy, lymph nodes along the trachea and upper esophagus as well as lymph nodes in the lateral compartment (i.e. deep external cervical and deep lateral cervical regions), are removed bilaterally.

## Minimally Invasive Esophagectomy

In an effort to limit the physiologic stress of esophagectomy while preserving the principle of en bloc resection, a minimally invasive approach to esophageal resection allowing the same type of resection compared to the transthoracic approach has been developed (Fig. 9.4).

The best indications for minimally invasive esophagectomy (MIE) are Barrett's high grade dysplasia or small tumors (T1a or eventually T1b without suspicious nodes). The patient is intubated with a single lumen tube and positioned supine in the jackknife position. The first port is placed in the right paramedian position after a $CO_2$ pneumoperitoneum is established to a pressure of 15 mmHg. The remaining four ports are placed under laparoscopic visualization.

The stomach is mobilized using the ultrasonic sheers and clips where necessary. Care is taken during this dissection to preserve the gastroepiploic arcade. With the greater and lesser curves mobilized, the stomach can be retracted superiorly allowing exposure of the left gastric vessels, and dissection of the left gastric and celiac axis lymph nodes. The vascular pedicle is divided with an endovascular stapler, most easily with the lesser curve exposure.

A narrow gastric tube is constructed by dividing the stomach starting at the distal lesser curve, following transection of the right gastric vessels. Careful, atraumatic construction of the gastric tube is critical. Every effort is made to minimize

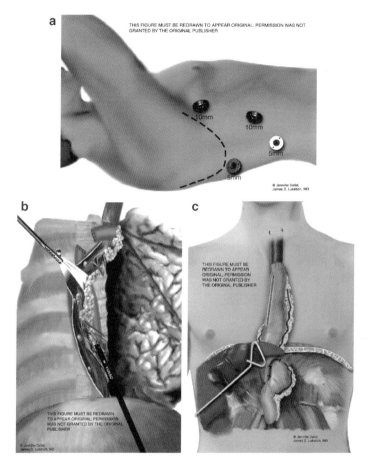

FIGURE 9.4. (a) Total thoracoscopic – laparoscopic esophagectomy. Position of the trocars. (b) Mobilization of the esophagus with division of azygos vein. (c) Completed reconstruction (Reprinted from Luketich, 2003 Copyright 2003 with permission of Annals of Surgery).

traumatic grasping of the stomach during the dissection. The gastric tube is then sutured to the stomach at the distal resection margin. The next step in the abdominal operation includes dissection of the phrenoesophageal ligament, which opens the plane into the thoracic cavity.

The patient is then intubated with a left-sided double lumen endotracheal tube and positioned in the full left lateral decubitus for right thoracoscopy; the right lung is deflated. Four thoracoscopic ports are introduced into the right hemithorax. The azygos vein is divided with an endovascular stapler. The esophagus is dissected circumferentially. Care is taken to avoid injury to the right or left main stem bronchi as the subcarinal nodes are removed en bloc with the specimen. During mobilization, thoracic duct lymphatic channels and aorto-esophageal vessels should be carefully divided. The dissection is carried superiorly into the thoracic inlet. Dissection of all mediastinal lymphatics including paraesophageal nodes, subcarinal nodes, nodes along the recurrent laryngeal nerve, and nodes along the brachiocephalic trunk up to the lower cervical lymph nodes is possible.

The esophagogastric specimen is then pulled up out through the left cervical incision and the anastomosis is fashioned in a separate cervical incision.

## The Debate: Lesser or More Radical Approach

Over the years, controversy remained as to the radicality of resection and extent of lymphadenectomy. Those who believe that lymph node involvement equates to systemic disease will advocate a simple resection and reconstruction, typically via a transhiatal approach.

Advocates of more radical surgery suggest that the natural course of the disease may be influenced in a positive way by radical esophagectomy and extensive (two-or three-field) lymphadenectomy typically performed through a transthoracic approach. Although several publications both from Japan and the West seem to indicate a benefit in favor of the more radical approach, definitive proof is lacking. More radical resections seem to result in overall survival rates between 35% to 50% (Table 9.1a), whereas transhiatal resection has 5-year survival rates between 15% to 20% (Table 9.1b), but

TABLE 9.1A.  Survival after radical surgery.

| Author | | N pat. | 3-year survival | 5-year survival |
|---|---|---|---|---|
| Ando | Ann Surg 2000 | 419 | 52% | 40% |
| Akiyama | Ann Surg 1994 | 913 | 52,6% | 42.40% |
| Isono | Oncology 1991 | 1,740 | 42% | 34.30% |
| JCOG9204 | JCO 2003 | 242 | 65% | 52% |
| Lerut | Ann Surg 2004 | 174 | 55% | 42% |
| Collard | Ann Surg 2001 | 235 R0 | 65% | 49% |
| | | 324 R0–R2 | 50% | 35% |
| Hagen | Ann Surg 2001 | 100 | 60% | 52% |
| Altorki | Ann Surg 2001 | 111 | 52% | 40% |
| Hulscher | NEJM 2002 | 114 | 42% | 40% |

TABLE 9.1B.  Survival after radical surgery, Stage III ($T_{3-4}N_1$).

| Author | | N pat. | 5-year survival |
|---|---|---|---|
| Ando | Ann Surg 2000 | 201 | 37.6 |
| Akiyama | Ann Surg 1994 | 175 | 27% (2F)/56% (3F) |
| Baba | Ann Surg 1994 | 22 | 30% |
| Lerut | J Thor Cardiovasc Surg | 162 | 26% |
| Collard | Ann Surg 2001 | 98 | 30% |
| Hagen | Ann Surg 2001 | 32 | 26% |
| Altorki | JTCVS 1997 | 33 | 34.5% (4 year) |

these non-randomized data may have been influenced by selection bias.

Hulscher et al. recently published a randomized trial comparing limited transhiatal resection versus transthoracic resection with extended en bloc lymph node dissection for adenocarcinoma of the esophagus and GEJ. Although no statistically significant overall difference was evident, there was a clear long-term trend in favor of the more extensive approach, in particular for adenocarcinoma of the distal esophagus. From the Japanese data and some series in Western centers, it seems that cervical lymphadenectomy (three-field) may offer a survival advantage for patients with supra-carinal tumors. In squamous cell carcinoma, Alkorki reported a 5-year survival of 40% and Lerut obtained for middle-third squamous cell carcinoma a 5-year survival of 28% following three-field lymphadenectomy in patients with positive cervical lymph node. These results definitively question the value of the actual UICC/TNM staging of these tumors in which cervical lymph node involvement is classified as Stage IV disease, and which is generally considered as a non-curable disease. Outcomes data further suggest the influence of hospital volume indicating the potential beneficial effect of centralization of esophagectomy as suggested by an increasing number of publications.

# Quality of Life After Operation

The intent of potentially curative resection and reconstruction in symptomatic esophageal cancer patients is improvement in their quality of life, even when the resection is only considered palliative. Both curative and palliative surgery improves food passage. The nature of the operation – transhiatal versus transthoracic, or the position of the proximal anastomosis - high thoracic versus cervical, provides only limited effect on the quality of life. Gastro-esophageal reflux and dumping syndrome are encountered in more than half of the patients. Twenty to 25% of patients also encounter problems ingesting solid food as a result of the relative stenosis of the proximal anastomosis. An anastomosis at the cervical level has a significantly lower probability of symptomatic reflux than one positioned within the thorax; however, the thorax anastomosis has a higher probability of leakage and benign stricturing. Global quality scores reveal a significant decrease in physical and role functional scales with an increase in fatigue, nausea, pain, dyspnea, deglutition, and GI symptoms. However, a gradual improvement is noticed over time; one year following resection, patients not suffering from tumor recurrence consider their quality of life comparable to that of their pre-disease state. Ten years after operation two-thirds of the surviving patients appear to maintain satisfactory ability for solid-food ingestion.

A disturbing finding at long term follow-up however is the development of metaplastic columnar mucosa in the cervical esophagus after esophagectomy. This most likely results as a consequence of acid and bile reflux. The true importance and risk for malignant degeneration of this observation is not yet known.

# Selected Readings

Akiyama H, Tsurumaru M, Kawamura T, Ono Y (1981) Principles of surgical treatment for carcinoma of the esophagus: analysis of lymph node involvement. Ann Surg 194:438–446

Akiyama H, Tsurumaru M, Udagawa H, Kajiyama Y (1994) Radical lymph node dissection for cancer of the thoracic esophagus. Ann Surg 220:364–373

Altorki N, Kent M, Ferrara C, Port J (2002) Three-field lymph node dissection for squamous cell and adenocarcinoma of the esophagus. Ann Surg 236:177–183

Belsey RH (1988) Surgical exposure of the esophagus. In: Skinner DBJ, Belsey RH (eds) Management of esophageal disorders. W.B. Saunders, Philadelphia, pp. 192–201

Birkmeyer JD, Siewers AE, Finlayson EV et al. (2002) Hospital volume and surgical mortality in the United States. N Engl J Med 346: 1128–1137

Clark GW, Peters JH, Ireland AP et al. (1994) Nodal metastasis and sites of recurrence after en bloc esophagectomy for adenocarcinoma. Ann Thorac Surg 58:646–654

Hulscher JB, van Sandlick JW, de Boer AG et al. (2002) Extended transthoracic resection compared with limited transhiatal resection for adenocarcinoma of the esophagus. N Engl J Med 347:1662–1669. See also N Engl J Med 2003, 348:1177–1174

Kato H, Watanabe H, Tachimori Y, Lizuka T (1991) Evaluation of neck lymph node dissection for thoracic esophageal carcinoma. Ann Thorac Surg 51:931–935

Lerut T, Nafteux P, Moons J et al. (2004) Three field lymphadenectomy for carcinoma of the esophagus and gas-troesophageal junction in 174 $R_0$ resections. Impact on staging, disease free survival and outcome. A plea for adaptation of the TNM classification in upperhalf esophageal carcinoma. Ann Surg 240:962–974

Lerut T, Van Lanschot J (2004) Cancer of the esophagus and gastro-esophageal junction: surgical aspects, Chapter 3. In: Van Lanschot J, Gouma D, Jansen P et al. (eds) Integrated medical and surgical gastroenterology. Bohn Stafleu Van Loghum, Houten, The Netherlands

Lewis I (1946) The surgical treatment of carcinoma of the esophagus with special reference to a new operation for growths of the middle third. Br J Surg 34:18–31

Logan A (1963) The surgical treatment of carcinoma of the esophagus and cardia. J Thorac Cardiovasc Surg 46:150–161

Luketich JD, Alvelo-Rivera M, Buenaventura PO et al. (2003) Minimally invasive esophagectomy: outcomes in 222 patients. Ann Surg 238: 486–494

McKeown KC (1976) Total three-stage esophagectomy for cancer of the esophagus. Br J Surg 63:259–262

McLarthy AJ, Deschamps C, Trastek VF et al. (1997) Esoophageal resection for cancer of the esophagus: long-term function and quality of life. Ann Thorac Surg 63:1568–1572

Oberg S, Johansson J, Wenner J, Walther B (2002) Metaplastic columnar mucosa in the cervical esophagus after esophagectomy. Ann Surg 235:338–345

Pearson FG (1995) Synchronous combined abdominothoraco-cervical esophagectomy, Chapter 42. In: Pearson FG, Deslauriers J, Ginsberg RJ et al. (eds) Esophageal surgery. Churchill Livingstone, New York

Skinner DB (1983) En bloc resection for neoplasms of the esophagus and cardia. J Thorac Cardiovasc Surg 65:59–71

Sweet RH (1945) Surgical management of carcinoma of the midthoracic esophagus. Preliminary report. N Engl J Med 433:1–7

# Part III
# Stomach: Benign and Malignant

# 10
# Peptic Ulcer Disease and Helicobacter Pylori

**Kent-Man Chu**

## Pearls and Pitfalls

- *Helicobacter pylori* plays a prominent role in upper gastro-intestinal disease worldwide.
- More than 50% of the world's population is infected with the organism; in those infected individuals, the estimated lifetime risk for ulcer disease and gastric cancer are 15% and 0.5–2%, respectively.
- Whether an individual will develop *H. pylori*-related disease depends on bacterial virulence, host genetic susceptibility, and environmental factors.
- There appears to be a negative association between *H. pylori* infection and gastroesophageal reflux disease.
- *H. pylori*-related duodenal and gastric ulcers are associated with antral-predominant and diffuse gastritis, respectively.
- Twenty percent of patients are asymptomatic until complications develop.
- First-line eradication treatment involves triple therapy with a proton pump inhibitor or ranitidine bismuth citrate, and two antimicrobial agents like clarithromycin, amoxicillin, or metronidazole. Medications are given twice daily for 7–14 days.
- In patients with perforated duodenal ulcer, when present, *H. pylori* is the most important factor associated with subsequent ulcer recurrence; eradication of *H. pylori*

K.I. Bland et al. (eds.), *Surgery of the Esophagus and Stomach*, DOI: 10.1007/978-1-84996-438-8_10,
© Springer-Verlag London Limited 2011

colonization is associated with a markedly reduced rate of ulcer recurrence.

- *H. pylori*-negative duodenal ulcer is independently associated with older age, concomitant medical problems, recent operation, underlying sepsis, and NSAID usage.
- *H. pylori*-negative duodenal ulcer presents more commonly with bleeding, with a larger ulcer, or with multiple ulcers.

## Introduction

Peptic ulcer disease is a global health problem. It has long been recognized that acid plays an important and necessary role in peptic ulcer disease, and reduction of acid production has been the primary goal in both medical and surgical treatment of the disease. Nevertheless, despite the introduction of potent acid-lowering medications, recurrence of ulcer has been frequent after cessation of medication.

The past two decades have seen profound changes in our understanding of peptic ulcer disease and with this knowledge have come marked changes in our approach toward treatment. There have been two major advances. First, minimally invasive surgical techniques were applied to elective operation for resistant ulcer disease as well as to emergency operation for ulcer perforation. Second, *Helicobacter pylori* was recognized as an important cause of ulcer disease after the bacteria was first described by Warren and Marshall in 1983. It is now possible to cure peptic ulcer disease in many patients by eradicating *H. pylori*.

Today, thanks to the success of ulcer treatment by eradication of *H. pylori* colonization, the need for elective operation of ulcer disease has decreased markedly or virtually disappeared. Nevertheless, ulcer complications and *H. pylori* negative ulcer disease remain prominent clinical problems, especially in our aging population.

# Helicobacter Pylori

## *The Organism*

*H. pylori* infection of the stomach is not a new phenomenon. As early as 1893, the Italian investigator Giulio Bizzozero described spiral organisms in the stomach. In 1915, Rosenow and Sanford described what they believed to be streptococci in the margins of gastric and duodenal ulcers. In 1938, Doenges reported finding spirochetes in 103 (43%) of 242 stomachs examined at autopsy, and in 1975, Steer reported gram-negative bacteria over the gastric mucosa in about 80% of patients with gastric ulcer. But it was not until 1983, when Warren and Marshall (both awarded the Nobel Prize in 2005) reported the successful culture of *"Campylobacter" pyloridis*, that the potential importance of this bacterium began to be appreciated. In 1989, the organism was renamed *Helicobacter pylori*. Since then, 18 other *Helicobacter* species have been found, one in man and the remainder in other animals.

*H. pylori* is a curved or S-shaped, gram-negative rod approximately 0.5 by 3 μm in size that is a microaerophilic, motile organism usually with four to seven sheathed flagella at one pole. The *H. pylori* genome consists of a single circular chromosome encoding about 1,600 genes. The unique characteristic of *H. pylori* is its ability to produce urease.

The natural habitat of *H. pylori* is the human stomach. The bacteria are found particularly on mucus-secreting cells because of strong and specific binding of bacteria to a protein, Trefoil factor 1, expressed by these cells. In an infected stomach, the highest density of *H. pylori* is found in the antrum. In the biopsy-based tests for *H. pylori*, therefore, biopsies should be obtained from the antrum to minimize sampling error. Interestingly, the greatest density of the-bacteria will shift to the proximal stomach after treatment with a potent acid inhibitor, like a proton pump inhibitor. The method of transmission or infection with *H. pylori* is not defined clearly, but current evidence is consistent with both oral-oral and fecal-oral transmission. Interpersonal transmission or infection from a single environmental source is suggested by studies showing an increased prevalence among family members of patients with *H. pylori* infection.

## Epidemiology

Studies of populations in developing countries suggest that, until the last century, nearly all humans carried *H. pylori* or closely related bacteria in their stomachs. *H. pylori* infection is usually acquired in childhood. With improvements in socio-economic conditions, fewer children are infected with *H. pylori*. Improvement in nutrition and a clean water supply have been proposed for this trend. Alternatively, some investigators have proposed that most transmission is from child to child and that decreasing family size reduces the chance for transmission. Currently, more than 50% of the world's population is infected with the organism. In addition, there is usually an increase in *H. pylori* prevalence with increasing age, suspected to be due to a cohort effect in which the greater prevalence in older individuals is the result of a greater rate of infection earlier in life.

On the whole, the prevalence of *H. pylori* infection is about 30–40% in the developed countries and 80–90% in the developing countries. In Asia, Malaysia has the lowest prevalence rate of about 5%, while most of the other Asian countries have a prevalence rate of about 60%.

## Disease Associations

Infection with *H. pylori* causes an element of histologic chronic gastritis in all those infected, but not all individuals with *H. pylori* infection will develop ulcer disease. In fact, the estimated lifetime risk for ulcer disease is only about 15%, a concept still imprecisely understood.

As many as 2% of individuals with *H. pylori* infection may develop gastric cancer. In 1994, *H. pylori* was declared a

Group 1 (a definite cause of cancer in humans) carcinogen by the International Agency for Research on Cancer (IARC) based on 13 epidemiologic studies reporting odds ratios between 2.13 and 8.67 of developing gastric cancer if infected by *H. pylori*. Chronic inflammation as a result of *H. pylori* infection can lead to gastric atrophy and intestinal metaplasia, a suspected precursor of gastric cancer. An experimental model of gastric cancer related to *H. pylori* infection has been developed in Mongolian gerbils. *H. pylori* infection also increases the risk of developing gastric mucosa-associated lymphoid tissue (MALT)lymphoma by six-fold; this association is important because the eradication of *H. pylori* alone may lead to regression of low grade MALT lymphomas.

Whether an individual will develop *H. pylori*-related disease appears to depend on three factors: virulence of the strain of *H. pylori*, host genetic susceptibility, and environmental factors such as diet and smoking. The most important bacterial virulence factors are related to the cytotoxin-associated gene(cagA) and vacuolating cytotoxin-associated gene (*vacA*). The *cagA* + strains induce more intense inflammation and are associated more commonly with ulcer disease and gastric cancer than are the cagA – strains. The high prevalence of *cagA* + strains in China and Japan appears to explain the greater incidence of gastric cancer in these countries. Unlike *cagA*, the *vacA* gene is present in all strains. *vacA* is, however, polymorphic, varying most notably in two regions called the mid-(m1 and m2) and signal (s1 and s2) regions. Among all the combinations, the s1m1 type of *vacA* is associated more commonly with duodenal ulcer and gastric cancer. The inflammatory response to *H. pylori* infection is dependent on the host genetics. Polymorphisms in the host cytokine genes influence the level of cytokine production by cells after contact with *H. pylori*. Polymorphisms in the IL-1β gene cluster are associated with an augmented cytokine response to *H. pylori*, which appears to increase the risk of gastric atrophy, achlorhydria, intestinal metaplasia, gastric ulcer, and gastric cancer.

The role of *H. pylori* infection in the development of gastroesophageal reflux disease (GERD) remains controversial.

It appears that *H. pylori* may protect against the development of GERD in some individuals. Reflux esophagitis and esophageal adenocarcinoma are rare in countries where *H. pylori* infection is common. The efficacy of proton pump inhibitors appears to be better in the presence of *H. pylori* infection.

An increasing number of extra-digestive conditions are associated with *H. pylori* infection. Examples include idiopathic thrombocytopenic purpura (ITP), coronary artery disease, bronchiectasis, cerebrovascular disease, growth retardation, diabetes mellitus, and auto-immune thyroiditis. Although an association with *H. pylori* infection has not been fully confirmed, the latest Maastricht Guidelines for *H. pylori* eradication developed by the European *Helicobacter pylori* Study Group (EHSG) recommend *H. pylori* eradication as the first line treatment for patients with ITP who are *H. pylori* positive.

# Pathogenesis of Ulcer Disease

Although genetic factors appear to be important from previous epidemiologic studies, it remains unclear how they contribute to the development of ulcer disease. The concordance for ulcer disease among identical twins is approximately 50%. About 40% of patients with duodenal ulcer have a positive family history. It is uncertain whether the apparently greater risk of ulcer disease in first-degree relatives can be explained by the transmission of *H. pylori* within families or by the host genetic susceptibility as explained above.

Although *H. pylori* is very important, no single pathogenic mechanism has been identified for ulcer disease. The pathogenesis of ulcer disease appears to be multifactorial and involves factors like acid secretion, mucosal defense, and environmental factors.

*Acid secretion*: The Schwarz's dictum "no acid – no ulcer" has been cited in textbooks since its first description in 1910 and appears to still be true. Prior to the discovery of *H. pylori*, three major disturbances in gastric physiology were noted in patients with duodenal ulcer disease: increased basal and stimulated acid secretion,impairedacidinhibitionofgastrinrele asefromtheantrum,andincreased acid load in the duodenum. Patients with duodenal ulcer produce on average twice the amount of gastric acid in response to the same degree of gastrin stimulation as patients who do not have a duodenal ulcer. This relative increase in acid secretion was postulated to be due to an increase in the mass of parietal (acid-secreting) cells in the stomach or to an increased sensitivity to circulating gastrin.

Duodenal ulcer only develops when *H. pylori*-related inflammation occurs predominantly in the antrum. Exactly how antral *H. pylori* leads to ulceration in the duodenal mucosa is not well understood and appears to be multifactorial. *H. pylori* infection of the antral mucosa results in depletion of antral somatostatin and an increased release of gastrin, and thus an increase in acid secretion. As a result of the prolonged exposure to acid, the duodenal mucosa will develop gastric metaplasia. *H. pylori* is able to then colonize this metaplastic mucosa and the resultant inflammation further precipitates duodenal ulcer formation.

Unlike duodenal ulcer, gastric ulcer is also associated with diffuse gastritis. *H. pylori*-related gastric ulcer is found most commonly at the transitional zone between antrum and corpus on the lesser curve. This region has a tendency for dense colonization of *H. pylori*, intense inflammation, and intestinal metaplasia, and the resultant epithelial damage leads directly to ulceration; how and why the ulcer develops here, however, is still not well understood.

*Mucosal defense*: Mucosal bicarbonate secretion, prostaglandin production, and blood flow are all important for mucosal defense. Although the gastric lumen is highly acidic, the production of mucus and bicarbonate by the mucosal cells maintains an almost neutral pH at the mucosal surface. A lower basal bicarbonate secretion occurs in patients with duodenal ulcer in comparison with normal individuals. Moreover, after instillation of a physiologic amount of hydrochloric acid, the bicarbonate secretion in patients with duodenal ulcer is only about 40% of the normal response. In such individuals, therefore, even if normal amounts of acid are produced, duodenal ulcer can still occur, because the bicarbonate secretion is lower than normal. Consistent with this concept is the observation that duodenal bicarbonate secretion returns to normal after eradication of *H. pylori* in patients with duodenal ulcer. In an animal study, *H. pylori* hinders duodenal nitric oxide synthase activity and subsequent bicarbonate secretion.

Reduction of mucosal prostaglandin production appears to be another contributing factor in ulcer formation. Prostaglandins stimulate the duodenal mucosa to secrete bicarbonate. In patients with duodenal ulcer, gastric mucosal production of prostaglandin E2 and other prostanoids is decreased.

Maintenance of gastric mucosal blood flow enhances mucosal defense. Apart from supplying nutrients and oxygen to the mucosal cells, mucosal blood flow removes protons from the interstitial fluid so as to maintain an almost neutral pH. Gastric mucosal ischemia is believed to contribute to gastric ulcer formation. Patients with gastric ulcer have a lesser mucosal blood flow along the lesser curve of the stomach where gastric ulcers occur. Moreover, blood flow in the base of an ulcer is less than that of the normal mucosa; in contrast, at the edge of a healing ulcer, blood flow is greater. Other factors are known to affect gastric mucosal blood flow. Examples include epidermal growth factor and dopaminergic agonists which have a protective effect on ethanol-induced mucosal injury by the enhancement of gastric blood flow.

*Environmental factors*: Environmental factors that contribute to development of ulcer disease include cigarette smoking, dietary habits, environmental stress, non-steroidal anti-inflammatory drugs (NSAID), and *H. pylori* infection.

A number of mechanisms have been postulated to explain the harmful effects of cigarette smoking, including stimulation of acid secretion, reduction in prostaglandin synthesis, enhancing pyloric incompetence, increasing duodenogastric bile reflux, and decreasing gastric mucosal blood flow.

Cigarette smoking also impairs ulcer healing and increases the risk of ulcer recurrence.

Although dietary habits and environmental stress are thought to be important etiologic factors in ulcer disease, consistent evidence supporting their importance is lacking. Change in dietary habits has not been shown to accelerate ulcer healing.

The mechanisms by which NSAIDs produce mucosal damage are not fully understood but appear to involve both direct topical injury and systemic effects. The direct effects include injury of the gastric mucosal cells by the acidity of NSAIDs, decrease in mucus secretion, inhibition of mucosal production of prostaglandins (and thus mucosal protective function), and interference with cell turnover. The ulcerogenic actions of NSAIDs appear largely to be caused by their systemic effects. Inhibition of cyclooxygenase with a resultant decrease in prostaglandin production, especially PGE1, PGE2, and PGI2, is thought to be the most important cause. NSAIDs inhibit both plasma and mucosal prostaglandin production in man. Because mucosal prostaglandin production plays an important role in normal mucosal defense, reduction in prostaglandin production increases the risk of ulcer formation. The risk of developing an ulcer with NSAID usage appears to be further increased by a past history of peptic ulcer disease, advancing age, increasing NSAID dosage, concurrent intake of corticosteroids, cigarette smoking, and alcohol intake.

## Clinical Presentations of Ulcer Disease

Epigastric pain or discomfort is the most frequent symptom of gastroduodenal ulcer disease. Other common but non-specific symptoms include anorexia, weight loss, nausea, fatty food intolerance, bloating, and belching. The mean age of patients with gastric ulcer is older than that for patients with duodenal ulcer. Based on symptoms alone, it is often impossible to distinguish between duodenal and gastric ulcers. There is also considerable overlap of symptoms between ulcer disease and non-ulcer dyspepsia. Moreover, approximately 20% of patients are asymptomatic until the ulcer progresses to complications such as bleeding or perforation.

In view of the non-specific nature of the symptoms of ulcer disease, accurate diagnosis depends on flexible endoscopy, which allows direct inspection and biopsy for histologic examination of gastric ulcer and for *H. pylori* infection. A double-contrast oral barium study is an alternative, but it is impossible to obtain a biopsy for histologic diagnosis during a barium study.

About 15–20% of patients with an active gastric or duodenal ulcer develop gross hemorrhage, and occult blood loss is more common. When an ulcer crater erodes into a major vessel, severe bleeding may occur (see Chapter 13). The most important tool for the investigation of upper gastrointestinal bleeding is flexible endoscopy. Endoscopy allows accurate localization of the site of bleeding as well as assessment of stigmata of recent hemorrhage. Therapeutic intervention with injection of epinephrine or thermocoagulation can be performed during the same procedure.

When an ulcer erodes through the full thickness of the gastric or duodenal wall, it may perforate or penetrate into surrounding structures. Ulcer perforation is less common than hemorrhage but more common than obstruction. Perforation occurs in about 5–10% of patients with active ulcer disease. The patient with ulcer perforation presents typically with sudden onset of severe abdominal pain, marked abdominal tenderness, and ileus. An erect chest radiograph reveals the presence of free air under the diaphragm in the majority of patients with ulcer perforation. The condition is associated with substantial mortality, especially in patients with concurrent medical illness, preoperative shock, or long-standing perforation of more than 24 h.

Gastric outlet obstruction results from impairment of antral motility as a consequence of acute inflammation and edema around an ulcer or more likely from mechanical obstruction due to scarring from a chronic ulcer. The former tends to resolve with conservative treatment, while the latter usually requires operative or endoscopic intervention. Obstruction develops in less than 5% of patients with ulcer disease, and more commonly with duodenal, pyloric, or prepyloric ulcer. The onset is insidious, and patients may present with nausea, vomiting, and abdominal distension.

## Diagnosis of *H. Pylori* Infection

A variety of tests are available for the diagnosis of *H. pylori* infection. Such tests can be classified into invasive and non-invasive tests. Invasive tests require endoscopic mucosal biopsies. The traditional invasive tests include histology, rapid urease test, and culture, while the traditional non-invasive tests include urea breath test and serology. Two biopsy specimens are adequate for an accurate histologic diagnosis of *H. pylori* infection. The reported sensitivity and specificity of histology are both about 90%. Histologic examination, however, is expensive and labor-intensive, and the result is not usually available on the same day. For outpatients, it is highly desirable and cost-effective to obtain the *H. pylori* status during the same endoscopy procedure, so that they do not have to return again for future investigation of appropriate treatment. The rapid urease test on gastric biopsy specimens is considered to be the initial test of choice in patients undergoing endoscopy because of its low cost, rapid availability of results, simplicity, and accuracy. This test involves a preparation containing urea and a pH sensitive marker. In the presence of urease produced by *H. pylori*, urea will be converted to ammonia with a resultant change in pH and thus in color. The CLO test (Delta West Ltd., Perth, Australia), which consists of an agar gel containing urea, phenol red, buffers and a bacteriostatic agent in a sealed plastic slide, was the first urease test to become available commercially. To date, several commercial kits are marketed for urease testing; all have good sensitivities (80–98%) and specificities (94–100%) for the diagnosis of *H. pylori* infection. A number of locally made, non-commercial preparations have also been described; these preparations are considerably cheaper than the commercial kits but are equally accurate for the diagnosis of *H. pylori* infection. The use of a rapid urease test to confirm successful eradication of *H. pylori* is not recommended because of the higher chance of false negative test as a result of a low density of bacteria.

Culture of *H. pylori* is difficult and accounts for its low sensitivity of 60–90%.Culture, however, is the most specific test (100%) for *H. pylori* infection. Culture is usually reserved for research studies or for testing of antibiotic sensitivity.

More sophisticated invasive tests include polymerase chain reaction (PCR) and confocal endomicroscopy. PCR will increase the detection rate of *H. pylori* in histologically negative biopsies. It can also be used to detect bacterial virulence factors like *cagA* and to assess antibiotics suscep-tibility. Confocal endomicroscopy allows direct observa-tion of bacteria in the gastric mucosa after topical application of acriflavine stain, but it is more cumbersome and expensive.

The urea breath test (UBT) is considered the best test for *H. pylori* after eradication therapy when repeated assessment by endoscopy is not necessary. The reported sensitivity and specificity are both about 95%. Two versions of UBT are available, one using non-radioactive 13C-urea and the other using radioactive 14C-urea. In the presence of *H. pylori*, the bacterial urease will convert the orally ingested labeled urea into ammonia and labeled carbon dioxide. The breath sample is then collected and analyzed. Although a simple test, the radioactive version is not recommended for pregnant women or children. The 13C-UBTrequiresa mass spectrometer for analysis and is, therefore, more expensive.

Serology is one of the least expensive tests for *H. pylori*. The sensitivity and specificity vary widely between different preparations. One major disadvantage of serology is its inability to differentiate between prior exposure and active infection. Several commercial stool antigen tests have become available in recent years. The available studies so far indicate that stool antigen tests are inferior to UBT, but they may be an alternative option when UBT is not available.

# Treatment of Ulcer Disease

*Medical treatment:* The earliest forms of medical treatment for ulcer disease involved dietary manipulation. The Sippy regimen introduced in 1915 (hourly feeding of milk and small bland meals), the Winkelstein milk drip introduced in the 1930s, the use of antacids and anticholinergic drugs, and bed rest were all considered standard treatment for ulcer disease until 40 years ago. Carbenoxolone sodium and other mucosal protective agents were introduced in the 1960s and 1970s. Owing to a lack of effective medication, operative treatment was considered the only effective long term means for preventing ulcer recurrence in the 1970s.

In the late 1970s, a large dose of antacid (equivalent to 1,000 mmol/day) was shown to result in healing of about 80% of duodenal ulcer after 4 weeks of treatment, confirming the therapeutic value of acid neutralization in ulcer healing. These large-dose antacid regimens were, however, inconvenient and tolerated poorly by patients.

Because defective mucosal defense was considered important in ulcer formation, mucosal protective agents like sucralfate and bismuth were introduced for the treatment of ulcer disease. In the 1970s, bismuth salts were demonstrated to be effective as a single agent in the healing of ulcer disease.

The discovery of the histamine H2-receptor antagonist cimetidine by Nobel laureate Sir James Black in 1972 marked an important milestone in the medical treatment of ulcer disease. The introduction of cimetidine coincided with the wide availability of flexible endoscopy and the general acceptance of the importance of prospective randomized, double blind, controlled trials for the assessment of treatment efficacy. More H2-receptor antagonists were developed subsequently, including ranitidine, famotidine, and nizatidine. The availability of the H2-receptor antagonists revolutionized the treatment of ulcer disease, and ulcer healing rates of 80–95% were attained after 6–8 weeks of treatment. Owing to their remarkable efficacy, good tolerability, ease of use, and excellent safety, H2-receptor antagonists were considered the standard treatment for ulcer disease throughout the 1980s.

The advent of proton pump inhibitor, omeprazole, achieved an even more powerful acid inhibition. Several other proton pump inhibitors, like esomeprazole, lansoprazole, pantoprazole and rabeprazole, are now available. These very potent acid inhibitors appear to produce more rapid ulcer healing than standard doses of H2-receptor antagonists. The intake of omeprazole 20 mg daily results in a duodenal ulcer healing rate of more than 90% after 4 weeks of treatment. Moreover, in several multi-center, double blind trials, omeprazole achieved significantly greater rates of duodenal ulcer healing at 2 weeks and, in most cases, at 4 weeks than H2-receptor antagonists.

Although the treatment of ulcer disease has been successful with the use of acid inhibitory drugs, ulcer recurrence after cessation of medication remains a problem. In fact, 50% of patients who received ranitidine alone for healing of duodenal or gastric ulcer suffered a relapse within 12 weeks of healing. In the past, either maintenance medical treatment or operative therapy was offered to such patients. Currently, a cure seems to be possible for patients with ulcer disease related to *H. pylori* infection.

*Eradication therapy*: In 1994, the National Institutes of Health Consensus Development Conference recommended the addition of antimicrobial agents to anti-secretory drugs to treat all patients with *H. pylori*-associated peptic ulcer disease. The development of effective therapies for the eradication of *H. pylori* has been difficult. Although the organism is sensitive to many antibiotics in vitro, the *in vivo* sensitivity is much less. In fact, none of the available antibiotics can achieve an eradication rate of more than 50% if given as a single agent. Borody and colleagues first described the "classical" triple therapy which consisted of bismuth, metronidazole, and tetracycline. Despite achieving an eradication rate of approximately 90% in meta-analysis, its success has been hindered by poor compliance, all-too-frequent side effects, and a decrease in efficacy with the development of metronidazole-resistant strains of *H. pylori*.

The first-line regimen today is triple therapy with a proton pump inhibitor or ranitidine bismuth citrate, and two antimicrobial agents like clarithromycin 500 mg, amoxicillin 1 g, or metronidazole 500 mg, all given twice daily for 7–14 days. The reported eradication rates vary owing to the different prevalence of drug-resistant strains among different populations. In general, the eradication rate is about 85–90%. In the case of eradication failure, culture and testing for antibiotics sensitivity should be considered. Quadruple therapy with bismuth 120 mg qid, a proton pump inhibitor bid, tetracycline 500 mg qid, and metronidazole 500 mg tid for 7 days is usually recommended. In a recent metaanalysis, the efficacy of a triple therapy containing levofloxacin for 10 days was superior to the classic quadruple therapy.

*Surgical treatment*: Historically, before the availability of anti-secretory drugs, the definitive treatment for ulcer disease was an operative anti-ulcer procedure. Theodor Billroth (1829–1894) performed the first successful distal gastrectomy for gastric cancer in 1881, followed shortly by a successful Billroth I gastrectomy by Ludwik Rydygier (1850–1920) for a benign pyloric ulcer. Rydygier also introduced gastrojejunostomy for the treatment of duodenal ulcer in 1884. Eugen Bircher (1882–1956) reported the performance of vagotomy. In 1922, Andre Latarjet (1876–1947) reported the need to add a drainage procedure, namely gastrojejunostomy, after a vagotomy.

During the 1920s, ulcers were generally thought to be due to gastric stasis, and the good results achieved by Latarjet were attributed to the gastrojejunostomy. It was not until the 1940s when Lester Dragstedt (1893–1975) established that a truncal vagotomy helps heal duodenal ulcers, because it decreases gastric secretion. Subsequently, the role of the antrum in gastric physiology became better understood, and vagotomy with antrectomy was recognized to reduce gastric acid secretion the best. In fact, the ulcer recurrence rate after this procedure is as low as 1%.

In the 1960s and 1970s, recognizing the side effects of truncal vagotomy, more selective types of vagotomy (selective vagotomy, proximal gastric vagotomy, and posterior truncal vagotomy with lesser curvature seromyotomy) were introduced. The more selective types of vagotomy, however, were associated with a somewhat higher ulcer recurrence rate of up to 30%.

The advent of laparoscopic surgery in the late 1980s was an important development in the history of ulcer surgery. With its advantages of a shorter and less painful post-operative course, shorter recovery times, earlier return to work, reduced scarring, and preservation of abdominal wall strength, laparoscopy has stimulated interest in transforming previously established open techniques into laparoscopic procedures. Laparoscopic anti-ulcer surgery was no exception. In fact, various laparoscopic acid-reduction procedures have been developed. While there was great excitement about the development of various laparoscopic procedures for peptic ulcer disease, the eradication of *H. pylori* became the established treatment for peptic ulcer disease in the early 1990s. As a result of the effectiveness of medical treatment, including eradication therapy for *H. pylori*, the need for elective operations for peptic ulcer disease have been almost eliminated in the recent decade.

Emergency operations are still required to treat ulcer complications like bleeding or perforation. The introduction of therapeutic endoscopy has diminished dramatically the need for emergency operation to treat bleeding peptic ulcers. Nevertheless, an emergency operation is indicated when endoscopic therapy fails. Currently, such elderly patients are often frail and have multiple medical problems.

## *H. Pylori* and Duodenal Ulcer Perforation

About 5–10% of patients with an untreated active duodenal ulcer will experience an episode of perforation during their lifetime. Closure with an omental patch remains standard treatment in many centers because of simplicity, short operating time, and low morbidity. In the past, simple closure was known to be associated with a very high rate of ulcer recurrence, 30–50%. Therefore, definitive acid reduction operations were advocated for emergency treatment of healthy patients with perforate duodenal ulcer in order to reduce the likelihood of recurrent ulceration. Recent studies, however, have shown that in younger patients with perforated duodenal ulcer, *H. pylori* is an important factor associated with subsequent ulcer recurrence, and its eradication is associated with minimal ulcer recurrence.

Currently, simple closure with an omental patch combined with intense antisecretory therapy for perforated duodenal ulcer is recommended. In the presence of irreversible pyloric stenosis, truncal vagotomy and pyloroplasty should be considered. Post-operatively, antisecretory drugs such as H2-receptor antagonists should be maintained until the *H. pylori* status is known. Gastroscopic examination should be performed 2 months after operation to both confirm healing of ulceration as well as to obtain antral biopsy specimens for determination of *H. pylori* status. Eradication therapy is recommended for patients who continue to test positive for *H. pylori*.

# *H. Pylori*-Negative Duodenal Ulcer Disease

Previous studies have reported that more than 90% of patients with duodenal ulcers and 60% with gastric ulcers are infected with *H. pylori*. The use of NSAIDs was suggested to be the major cause of duodenal ulcers in patients > 50 years old and in the remaining *H. pylori*-negative ulcer disease. The prevalence of *H. pylori* infection in patients with duodenal ulcer was believed to be so high that confirmatory testing before eradication treatment was considered unnecessary by some centers. Recently, however, the prevalence of *H. pylori*-positive duodenal ulcer was found to be decreasing and was only about 75% in a number of studies. It is therefore important to confirm the *H. pylori* status before prescribing eradication therapy.

*H. pylori*-negative duodenal ulcer was found to be associated independently with older age, concomitant medical problems, recent operation, underlying sepsis, and NSAID usage. It is noteworthy that *H. pylori*-negative duodenal ulcers present more commonly with bleeding, with a larger ulcer, or with multiple ulcers. In the elderly patient requiring emergency operation for bleeding duodenal ulcer, which is usually large in size, acid-reduction operation should be entertained in view of the likelihood that the ulcer is unrelated to *H. pylori* infection.

## Selected Readings

Chu KM, Kwok KF, Law SYK et al. (1999) *Helicobacter pylori* status and endoscopy follow-up of patients having a past history of perforated duodenal ulcer. Gastrointest Endosc 50:58–62

Chu KM, Kwok KF, Law S, Wong KH (2005) Patients with *Helicobacter pylori* positive and negative duodenal ulcers have distinct clinical characteristics. World J Gastroenterol 11:3518–3522

Marshall B (1983) Unidentified curved bacilli on gastric epithelium in active chronic gastritis. Lancet 1:1273–1275

McColl KEL (1997) Pathophysiology of duodenal ulcer disease. Eur J Gastroenterol Hepatol 9 (Suppl 1):S9–S12

Peterson WL, Fendrick AM, Cave DR et al. (2000) *Helicobacter pylori*-related disease: guidelines for testing and treatment. Arch Intern Med 160:1285–1291

Walsh JH, Peterson WL (1995) The treatment of *Helicobacter pylori* infection in the management of peptic ulcer disease. N Engl J Med 333:984–991

Warren JR (1983) Unidentified curved bacilli on gastric epithelium in active chronic gastritis. Lancet 1:1273

# 11
# Peptic Ulcer Disease: Perforation

**Anja Schaible and Peter Kienle**

## Pearls and Pitfalls

- The epidemiology of peptic ulcer disease has changed dramatically
- The medical management of symptomatic peptic ulcer disease has improved
- There has been no decrease in ulcer perforations over the last decades
- Two main trends responsible for the unchanged rate of complications (perforation, bleeding)
- Decrease in prevalence of *Helicobacter pylori*
- Increase in use of NSAIDs
- Ulcer perforations occur mostly in stomach (60%) or duodenum (40%)
- One third to one half of ulcer perforations are associated with NSAID use
- Clinical presentation tends to occur in 3 phases

    - Phase one: 0–2 h after onset, Initial sudden onset of severe abdominal pain
    - Phase two: 2–12 h after onset, Less abdominal pain
    - Phase three: >12 h after onset, Increasing abdominal extension

- Rapid diagnosis is essential!
- Perforation is largely a clinical diagnosis: abdominal rigidity

K.I. Bland et al. (eds.), *Surgery of the Esophagus and Stomach*, DOI: 10.1007/978-1-84996-438-8_11,
© Springer-Verlag London Limited 2011

- Abdominal x-ray: look for free air; no further examination necessary: this is an indication for surgical exploration
- Basic support involves: intravenous fluid, nasogastric tube, antibiotics
- Further therapy

  - Non operative management is possible in selected patients
  - Normally: surgical exploration, is indicated, possibly laparoscopic

    Prompt closure or patching with omentum of the site of perforation
    Lavage with 10–20 l

- Morbidity and mortality have decreased
- Mortality rate for operations after peptic ulcer perforation, however, remains high at 2–8%

# Introduction

The epidemiology of peptic ulcer disease continues to change. Ulcer incidence increases with age for both duodenal and gastric ulcers. Duodenal ulcers occur generally two decades earlier than gastric ulcers. All over the world, the incidence of ulcer has decreased over the last decades, more for duodenal ulcers than for gastric ulcers, and the overall frequency of hospitalization and death from peptic ulcer has diminished considerably. Despite dramatic improvements in the medical management (Proton Pump Inhibitors, PPI) and the lower rate of peptic ulcer disease, the incidence of potentially life-threatening ulcer complications such as perforation (and bleeding) has not decreased over the last decades.

Two opposing main trends are responsible for the stable complication rate: first a decrease in the prevalence of *Helicobacter pylori* due to improved socioeconomic conditions, and second, an increase in use of non steroidal antiinflammatory drugs (NSAID). NSAID use, which is an independent risk factor for ulcers, is common especially in elder individuals.

These two main trends have resulted in an increase in ulcer complications in older patients and a decline in younger patients. There are not much data regarding the frequency of complications but suggest that complications occur at a rate of 1–2% per ulcer per year. Giant ulcers and pyloric channel ulcers may be associated with a higher rate of complications. The majority of gastric ulcers are located along the lesser curvature and anterior wall especially in the antrum, whereas duodenal ulcers are localized predominantly in the first part of the duodenum, especially on the anterior surface. Seldom, perforations are located on the dorsal wall toward the lesser omentum.

Ulcer perforations due to peptic ulcer disease are located mostly in the stomach or duodenum. Other small intestinal ulcers are defined as defects in the gastrointestinal mucosa extending through the muscularis mucosa and can generally occur in the whole gastrointestinal tract. Other organs are affected only rarely and should be distinguished from peptic (acid-induced) ulcers, e.g. ulcers in the proximal small bowel from drug exposure, or especially after oral potassium chloride tablets, NSAIDs or aspirin, or in the wake of blood flow disturbances or in the postoperative setting. Advanced malignant diseases seldom show free perforation of the tumor. Important causes for peptic ulcers are listed in Table 11.1.

Duodenal and gastric ulcers account for 60% and 40% of perforations due to peptic ulcer disease. One third to one half of perforated ulcers are associated with NSAID use; these usually occur in elderly patients. Low dose aspirin increases the risk of GI complications caused by NSAIDs and selective Cox-2 inhibitors. The association between ulcer perforation and *H. pylori* remains controversial: some studies found a correlation, while others did not.

## Clinical Presentation

Peptic ulcers may present with a wide variety of symptoms. Although many patients complain of upper abdominal discomfort, others are completely asymptomatic, sometimes

TABLE 11.1. Important causes for gastrointestinal ulcers.

| Note | |
| --- | --- |
| Infection | *Helicobacter pylori* |
| | HSV |
| | CMV |
| Drug exposure | NSAIDs |
| | Aspirin |
| | Corticosteroids |
| | Bisphosphonates |
| | Clopidogrel |
| | Potassium chloride |
| | Chemotherapy |
| Hormonal or mediator-induced | Gastrinoma (Zollinger-Ellison syndrome) |
| | Systemic mastocytosis |
| | Antral G cell hyperfunction |
| Radiation therapy | |
| Infiltrating disease | Sarcoidosis |
| | Crohn's disease |
| Ulcer associated with systemic disease | Stress (ICU) ulcers |
| | Organ transplantation |

until perforation occurs. About one third of patients with peptic ulcer disease present with a complication as the first symptom, especially older individuals with NSAID-induced perforation. The majority of patients with peptic ulcer perforation, however, will have a history of ulcer symptoms.

In 1997, Silen described three clinical phases of perforated ulcer (see Table 11.2). In the initial phase (within 2 h of onset), patients develop sudden onset of severe abdominal pain, sometimes even producing syncope. Patients often

TABLE 11.2. Clinical phases of perforated ulcer.

| | |
|---|---|
| Phase 1 | 0–2 h after onset, Sudden severe abdominal pain |
| Phase 2 | 2–12 h after onset, Less pain than in phase 1 |
| Phase 3 | >12 h after onset, Increasing abdominal extension |

describe an abrupt pain like a thrust with a stab. Localization is usually epigastric, but it quickly becomes generalized and presents as an acute abdomen. Acid fluid in the peritoneal cavity releases vasoactive mediators causing tachycardia, cool extremities, and a low temperature. The severity of onset depends on how much fluid is released. The stage may last only a few minutes up to 2 h. Pain may radiate to the top of the right or both shoulders. Abdominal rigidity then begins to develop.

In the second phase, abdominal pain may lessen and may result in an underestimation of the situation. Patients in this phase often feel that things are getting better. Pain is usually less than in phase one but is now more generalized, often getting worse with movement. Rectal examination is often tender as is palpation of the right lower quadrant due to irritation from inflammatory fluid. The duration of the second phase is usually 2–12 h after primary onset.

The third phase usually begins more than 12 h after onset. Now increasing abdominal distension is noted, but abdominal pain, tenderness, and rigidity maybe less evident than in phase one. Temperature and hypovolemia due to third-spacing develop, tachycardia worsens, and hypovolemic shock may occur. The patient now looks very ill clinically, and rapid diagnosis is essential.

Not all patients develop the classic symptoms described above. Especially if patients have had abdominal operations previously with subsequent adhesions, the ulcer may not perforate into the free abdominal cavity but into other organs or be contained by the omentum. Therefore, patients with milder symptoms have to be evaluated carefully in order to exclude a perforation.

# Diagnosis

A detailed history should ask for ulcer symptoms in the last weeks such as abdominal pain especially in the epigastrium (Table 11.3). Abdominal pain before oral intake is associated with a duodenal ulcer, whereas pain after oral intake is more typical for a gastric ulcer. A prolonged ulcer history is common among patients with complicated ulcers; these patients with a history of complicated ulcer disease are prone to experiencing another complication. A detailed drug history in regard to NSAIDs, aspirin, corticosteroids, potassium chloride, and other drugs is mandatory.

Physical examination reveals exquisite tenderness, abdominal rigidity in all four quadrants per-haps accentuated in the epigastric area, rebound, and loss of bowel sounds. Physical examination provides the essential clues, because perforation is largely a clinical diagnosis.

In the diagnostic pathway, the next step is a blood sample for measuring leucocytes and CRP. An upright abdominal x-ray will show free air beneath the diaphragms (Fig. 11.1). If so, no further diagnostic studies are necessary, and an indication for operative exploration is present. In contrast, 10–20% of patients with an ulcer perforation will not have free air. In this situation, leakage of water soluble contrast (Gastrografin) is a useful confirmatory test. A better alternative is a CT with oral contrast in order to detect small amounts of free air or fluid. CT is able to detect both ulcer perforation and other pathologies such as colon perforation.

If the diagnosis remains unclear, an endoscopy of the stomach can help to make the diagnosis of perforation and is

TABLE 11.3. Diagnostic pathway.

| 1. Detailed history | Epigastric abdominal pain? |
| | Drugs (NSAIDs, aspirin)? |
| 2. Physical examination | Abdominal rigidity? Bowel movements? |
| 3. Blood sample | Leucocytes, CRP |
| 4. Abdominal x-ray | Free air? |

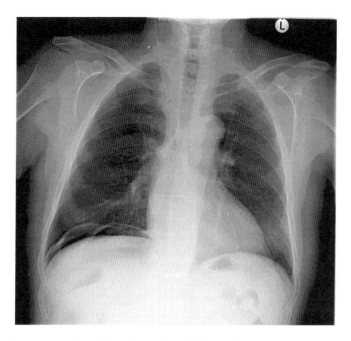

FIGURE 11.1. Note free air under right hemidiaphragm on upright chest radiograph.

not contraindicated in our opinion, although some groups believe so. Furthermore, endoscopy can localize the perforation and influence the operative procedure (laparoscopic or conventional approach).

For differential diagnosis, other etiologies of an acute abdomens have to be considered. First, other areas of potential of perforation must be considered, especially the sigmoid. But if there is free air in the x-ray, the patient usually requires operative intervention anyway, and exploration will show the location of the perforation. In contrast, there are a lot of other diseases which can cause an acute abdomen, such as perforated appendicitis, small bowel ileus or intussusception, acute pancreatitis, mesenterial infarction, and myocardial infarction (Table 11.4).

TABLE 11.4. Differential diagnosis of acute abdomen.

| |
|---|
| Appendicitis, acute or perforated |
| Small bowel intussusception or ileus |
| Perforated diverticulitis |
| Acute or perforated cholecystitis |
| Acute pancreatitis |
| Mesenterial infarction |
| Myocardial infarction |

## Treatment

Intravenous fluids, stabilization of hemodynamic instability, and nasogastric suction are the first steps of the treatment strategy, which have to be applied early on. The further treatment is operative, normally. Intravenous antibiotics should be administered prior to incision and when peritonitis is confirmed for up to 5 days postoperatively.

Nonoperative management, including parenteral nutrition and antibiotics, may be successful in well-selected patients. In 1989, Crofts et al. reported a group of 83 patients with a perforated ulcer randomized to initial medical therapy or immediate laparotomy with operative repair. In this study, 70% of the patients randomized to a nonoperative approach avoided operative intervention, while only 11 of 40 patients required surgery. The hospital stay was 35% longer in the group treated conservatively. The authors concluded that an initial period of non operative treatment with careful observation was safe in patients under age 70. When non operative management is considered, one has to be certain that no extravasation of contrast to the abdominal cavity occurs. Another possibility for non operative management is the unusual situation, where perforation is detected several days after the incident. Although some patients will seal their perforated ulcers without an operation, such an approach has been associated with morbidity and mortality, particularly in high-risk patients.

Normally, if clinical examination reveals abdominal rigidity, and free air is detected by x-ray or CT scan, operative intervention is generally required. A delay in intervention will be associated with a subsequent septic complication. The objective of therapy for perforation is prompt closure of the perforation in the duodenum or stomach. In the stomach, ulcers should be excised to rule out a malignancy, while in the duodenum, closure without excision is the usual practice. Usually, sutures placed in seromuscular fashion across the site of perforation are sufficient for secure closure. Some groups tie in a tag of omentum with these sutures to prevent a leakage of the suture line, but there is little evidence for this. Thorough lavage of the peritoneal cavity with 10–20 l fluid is an essential part of the operation.

Laparoscopic repair appears to be a reasonable option for patients with a history less than 24 h, with no hypovolemic shock, and with a perforation not more than 6 mm. In up to 25%, conversion to an open operation is necessary. Morbidity and mortality seem to be comparable in published series, but larger randomized studies are still lacking.

The role of definitive ulcer surgery with an acid-reducing procedure remains unclear without current understanding of ulcer pathogenesis. Most large studies of patients who have undergone definitive ulcer surgery were performed prior to the recognition of the role of *H. pylori* treatment. A recent randomized study showed that 1 year after a prompt closure and consequent *H. pylori* eradication, only 5% of patients developed recurrent ulcers. Therefore, our approach in most perforations is prompt closure with additional removal of the ulcer when localized in the stomach and an extensive lavage of the abdominal cavity. In selected cases of large perforating ulcers of the stomach, more extensive resections such as Billroth I or II resections may become necessary.

## Outcome

Morbidity and mortality after peptic ulcer perforation has decreased continuously over the last decades because of better antibiotic therapy. The main risk factors for mortality are the duration of the interval between perforation and operation, the patient's age, and comorbidity factors. In recent studies the mortality rate for operations after peptic ulcer perforation ranged between 2 to 8%.

## Selected Readings

Bloom BS, Kroch E (1993) Time trends in peptic ulcer disease and in gastritis and in duodenitis: mortality, utilization and disability in the United States. J Clin Gastoenterol 17:33–342

Crofts TJ, Park KG, Steele RJ et al. (1989) A randomized trial of non operative treatment for perforated peptic ulcer. N Engl J Med 320:970

El-Serag HB, Sonnenberg A (1998) Opposing time trends of peptic ulcer and reflux disease. Gut 43:327–33

Gunshefski L, Flancbaum L, Brolin RE, Frankel A (1990) Changing patterns in perforated peptic ulcer disease. Am Surg 56:270

Katkhouda N, Mavor E, Mason RJ et al. (1999) Laparoscopic repair of perforated duodenal ulcers: outcome and efficacy in 30 consecutive patients. Arch Surg 134:845–848

Ng EK, Lam YH, Sung JJ (2000) Eradication of Helicobacter pylori prevents recurrence of ulcer after simple closure of duodenal ulcer perforation: randomized controlled trial. Ann Surg 231:153–158

Silen W (1996) Cope's early diagnosis of the acute abdomen. Oxford University Press, New York

# 12
# Peptic Ulcer Disease: Obstruction

**David A. Berg and Daniel T. Dempsey**

## Pearls and Pitfalls

- The most common cause of gastric outlet obstruction in today's era of histamine receptor blockers, proton pump inhibitors, and effective treatment of *Helicobacter pylori* is malignancy, no longer peptic ulcer disease.
- Over 90% of serious peptic ulcer complications are associated with *Helicobacter pylori* infection, NSAID use, and/or smoking.
- The classic indications for operative intervention for peptic ulcer disease are perforation, bleeding, and obstruction; the latter is the least common.
- The primary symptom of gastric outlet obstruction is postprandial, non-bilious vomiting.
- Volume contraction and persistent vomiting of gastric contents leads to a hypochloremic, hypokalemic metabolic alkalosis in patients with gastric outlet obstruction.
- All patients with gastric outlet obstruction should have flexible upper endoscopy with biopsies of the stenosis and any active ulcer and/or scar. Upper GI contrast radiography often yields complimentary information.
- Gastric outlet obstruction from chronic peptic ulcer disease is unlikely to respond to conservative management and will require either endoscopic and/or operative intervention.

K.I. Bland et al. (eds.), *Surgery of the Esophagus and Stomach*, DOI: 10.1007/978-1-84996-438-8_12, © Springer-Verlag London Limited 2011

- An acute prepyloric or duodenal ulcer may cause gastric outlet obstruction due to edema and/or motor dysfunction; this usually resolves with gastric decompression and aggressive medical treatment.
- Endoscopic balloon dilation is a non-operative approach that offers excellent initial symptomatic relief in many patients with obstructing peptic ulcer, but the beneficial effect is often transient.
- More than two or three endoscopic dilations over greater than1year suggests that an operation should be considered to treat the obstruction from chronic peptic ulcer. Younger, good-risk patients should be considered for operation sooner.
- The operative procedures of choice for obstructing duodenal ulcer are highly selective vagotomy with gastrojejunostomy, and truncal vagotomy and antrectomy. The latter should be avoided in poor-risk or chronically asthenic patients and patients with a difficult duodenum.
- Obstruction associated with gastric ulcer (prepyloric or otherwise) is best treated with resection if this can be done safely. If resection is not performed, intraoperative biopsies should be considered.
- Pyloroplasty should be avoided as a drainage procedure in patients with obstructing peptic ulcer disease.

# Introduction

Fifty years ago, peptic ulcer was a surgical disease: operation was the only widely effective curative treatment. Currently, many clinicians view peptic ulcer as a non-operative disease. But this is not entirely accurate because the number of operations performed today for peptic ulcer complications (bleeding, perforation, obstruction) is similar to what it was 50years ago. Advances in the understanding of peptic ulcer pathophysiology and the development of more effective diagnostic and therapeutic modalities have decreased dramatically the number of operations performed electively for intractable, nonhealing peptic ulcers and for bleeding peptic ulcers. But there persists a subset of patients who develop life-threatening complications of peptic ulcer disease, namely recurrent or persistent bleeding, perforation, or obstruction, who will require operation for definitive treatment. It is essential that the general surgeon be familiar with the surgical options useful for the management of these complications. Herein, we present a brief overview of peptic ulcer disease, focusing specifically on management of gastric outlet obstruction. Approximately 2,000 patients per year will ultimately require operation for obstructing peptic ulcer disease.

# Causes of Gastric Outlet Obstruction in the Adult

Today the most common cause of gastric outlet obstruction is cancer, and not peptic ulcer disease. Thus, it is more important than ever for the surgeon not to mistake a malignant gastric outlet obstruction for a benign obstruction associated with peptic ulcer disease. The most likely primary adenocarcinomas presenting with gastric outlet obstruction are pancreatic, gastric, and duodenal in declining order of frequency. Primary lymphoma of the stomach, duodenum, or pancreas may also obstruct the gastric outlet; the same is true for GI stromal neoplasms of the stomach and duodenum. Extrinsic neoplastic obstruction of the gastric outlet may occur from metastatic disease to the porta hepatis. Rarely, recurrent colon cancer at the site of a previous ileocolonic anastomosis can obstruct the gastric outlet by direct extension.

Although several decades ago peptic ulcer disease was the most common cause of gastric outlet obstruction in adults, currently it is less common than obstruction due to cancer of the pancreas, stomach, or duodenum. Patients with obstructing peptic ulcer disease may have a long history of ulcer symptoms, but some have little or no history suggestive of chronic ulcer disease. The site of the primary ulcer maybe duodenal, gastric (type3-prepyloric, nottype 1-angularis, ortype

4-juxtaesophageal), or both (so called type 2-gastric ulcer). Commonly, there is a discrete stricture in the duodenal bulb, but other patterns are not uncommon, e.g. a prepyloric stricture, a post bulbar stricture, or a long chronic cicatrix extending from the prepyloric to postpyloric region.

Other possible benign causes of gastric outlet obstruction in the adult include entities that usually present in childhood such as duodenal web, duodenal duplication, and hypertrophic pyloric stenosis. Finally, it is important to consider primary gastroparesis or chronic bowel obstruction masquerading clinically as a mechanical gastric outlet obstruction, especially after a previous vagotomy.

## Pertinent Pathophysiology

Peptic ulcers form as a result of acid-peptic injury to the gastroduodenal mucosal barrier. *Helicobacter pylori* infection, NSAID use, and smoking are causative factors in the majority of duodenal and gastric ulcers, and over 90% of serious peptic ulcer complications are associated with one or more of these three factors. For the surgeon treating the patient with obstructing peptic ulcer, it is important to keep this in mind for several reasons. First, if the patient has gastric outlet obstruction from an acute edematous process, the blockage (mechanical and/or functional) may resolve with acid suppression and elimination of the causative factors. Although many patients with obstructing peptic ulcer will not have demonstrable *H. pylori* infection (i.e. the tests for helicobacter are negative), we treat this empirically whenever possible in all patients with ulcer disease severe enough to warrant surgical consultation. Second, the likelihood of recurrent or persistent ulcer after an operation for obstruction is dependent on the ability of the clinician and the patient to eliminate the associated causative factors. Thus it may be irrational to do a larger ulcer operation (e.g. vagotomy and antrectomy) in order to minimize the risk of recurrence if the surgeon is confident that the helicobacter, NSAIDs, and/or smoking can be eradicated. Finally, an absence of these causative factors should increase the index of suspicion for cancer or gastrinoma. Regarding the diagnosis of the latter, it is important to remember that antral distention is a stimulus for gastrin secretion. Thus it is not uncommon for the patient with obstructing peptic ulcer to have a somewhat increased serum gastrin level and gastric acid hypersecretion. A secretin stimulation test may be useful to rule out gastrinoma.

Chronic gastric outlet obstruction leads to gastric dilation, muscular hypertrophy, and abnormal gastric motor activity. Although surgical lore has suggested that the motor activity may improve after several days of gastric decompression, in our experience it may take weeks for gastric motor function to improve after operation for obstruction. If gastrojejunostomy is chosen as a surgical option to treat obstructing peptic ulcer, it is important to consider vagotomy, because the aforementioned acid hypersecretion may predispose to marginal ulceration. Motor function of the distal stomach (and therefore gastric emptying) may be better preserved if a highly selective vagotomy is performed rather than a truncal vagotomy. Rarely, gastrojejunostomy alone and lifelong proton pump inhibitors may be acceptable treatment in the selected, elderly but reliable patient. Last, it is important for the operating surgeon to be aware of the degree to which the gastric wall may thicken. Due to this strong consideration should be given to using the larger (i.e. green) stapling cartridges or to hand-sewing anastomosis and oversewing staple lines.

# Clinical Presentation of Obstructing Peptic Ulcer Disease

Patients with gastric outlet obstruction often present with a prolonged history of symptoms. The majority of patients complain of nausea relieved frequently by *nonbilious vomiting*. Abdominal distention or bloating, vague epigastric discomfort, early satiety, and/or weight loss are also common. Emesis of undigested food may occur as long as 24–48 h after ingestion. Not uncommonly, patients have eliminated many solid foods from their diets and often do not present to hospital until they are weakened acutely with dehydration. Physical examination may reveal epigastric tenderness, abdominal distension with or without tympany, hypoactive bowel sounds, or visible peristalsis. The classic sign of gastric outlet obstruction, a succussion splash, is present in only 25% of patients. Placing the stethoscope over the epigastrium and gently rocking the supine patient from side to side may elicit this sign. Volume contraction and electrolyte disturbances are common due to a prolonged history of nonbilious vomiting. The classic electrolyte abnormality is hypochloremic, hypokalemic, metabolic alkalosis. In chronic cases, patients may be severely malnourished, and parenteral nutrition should be considered.

Patients with obstructing peptic ulcer disease often report a history of previous ulcers, as well as the use of NSAIDs, antacids, or antisecretory drugs. Over 90% of patients report a recent or remote history of epigastric pain, often non-radiating and burning in character. Heme-positive stool and/ or anemia are not uncommon, but the latter may not be apparent until after rehydration.

## Diagnosis and Management

Peripheral intravenous access is established and fluid/electrolyte repletion begun with isotonic saline. A Foley catheter is placed. Once there is evidence of adequate renal function, potassium chloride is added to the intravenous solution. Vital signs, urine output, and electrolytes are followed as guides to the adequacy of resuscitation. Placement of a large bore nasogastric tube will decompress the stomach. Ideally, a plain upright x-ray of the chest and abdomen obtained prior to the placement of the tube often shows massive gastric distention with a large air fluid level; the absence of small bowel distention should corroborate the diagnosis of gastric outlet obstruction. The patient is maintained with nothing by mouth on nasogastric suction, and continuous intravenous proton pump inhibitors are administered. NSAIDs are eliminated if possible. Parenteral nutrition may be necessary. Once the patient has been resuscitated adequately and the stomach has been adequately decompressed, upper endoscopy is performed. It is imperative that biopsies of ulcers as well as the site of obstruction are performed to help rule out malignancy. A high index of suspicion for malignancy must exist especially in older patients and those without a known history of peptic ulcer disease. Age greater than 55 and lack of a history of peptic ulcer disease have been identified as independent predictors of malignant gastric outlet obstruction (up to a fivefold increased risk). Biopsies of the antrum are helpful in evaluating the presence of H pylori infection. An upper GI contrast study complements the upper endoscopy and is particularly useful to the surgeon in evaluating the anatomy of the antrum, pylorus, and duodenum. Abdominal CT should be considered if malignancy is suspected.

Numerous diagnostic criteria have been used to define gastric outlet obstruction. These criteria may include any of the following: postcibal gastric volume greater than 300 ml after 4 h, an overnight residual gastric volume greater than 200 ml, a positive saline load test (750 ml test volume with residual greater than 400 ml after 30 min), endoscopy revealing a stenotic pylorus preventing passage of a 9 mm endoscope, or an upper gastrointestinal contrast study with greater than 60% of barium retained in the stomach after 4 h. Most patients with benign gastric outlet obstruction secondary to peptic ulcer disease are managed clinically, with invasive treatment (endoscopic dilation or operation) reserved for patients who cannot tolerate a full liquid diet after about 1 week of intensive pharmacologic treatment and nasogastric decompression. Acute ulcers, often associated with clinically significant obstruction secondary to edema and/or impaired gastric motility, will usually respond to a 3–5 day conservative trial of hydration, decompression, and antisecretory therapy. Due to extensive pyloric scarring and rigidity, chronic gastric outlet obstructions from recurrent peptic ulcers are much less likely to respond to conservative management and will require either endoscopic and/or operative intervention.

At least 50% of patients admitted to hospital today with obstructing peptic ulcer will require such intervention.

## Endoscopic Balloon Dilation

Endoscopic balloon dilation is a non-operative approach that offers excellent initial symptomatic relief in many patients, but the beneficial effect is often transient. It is most useful in poor risk patients, or as a temporizing measure in patients with other active medical issues that make operation risky (e.g. recent myocardial infarction or active pneumonia). Endoscopic balloon dilation for peptic ulcer strictures has rendered both operative dilation and operative stricturoplasty for this disorder moot.

In studies with longer duration of follow-up, many patients (over 80% in some studies) eventually need repeated dilations, with a substantial proportion of those patients requiring operative treatment. Thus operation should be considered in most good-risk patients who fail conventional medical therapy. To date, large studies examining the long-term effects of endoscopic balloon dilation are lacking. No studies exist with median follow up greater than 4 years and sample size greater than 50 patients. Up to one half of patients requiring repeated dilatation for recurrent obstruction will require an operation ultimately. Factors shown to be predictive of requiring operative treatment are duration of endoscopic treatment greater than 1 year and the need for more than two or three endoscopic dilatations. Prior NSAID use, presence of an acute ulcer, site of obstruction, or gender does not influence the need for operative treatment after endoscopic dilatation.

The role of *Helicobacter pylori* in patients with benign gastric outlet obstruction treated with pneumatic dilatation is poorly defined. It has been speculated that effective treatment of *Helicobacter pylori* in patients with obstructing peptic ulcer disease will improve the outcome of balloon dilatation. Some gastroenterologists suggest that treatment of confirmed *Helicobacter pylori* infection is an important adjunct to endoscopic balloon dilatation if operation is to be avoided. Limited data show that patients negative for *Helicobacter pylori* respond poorly to endoscopic dilatation and should be considered for early surgical referral. Clearly, more data are needed to elucidate further the role that treatment of *Helicobacter pylori* may or may not play in the response to endoscopic balloon dilatation.

Endoscopic balloon dilatation for obstructing peptic ulcer was first reported in the early 1980s. Currently, a through-the-scope technique is used in which balloons of increasing diameters (8 mm through 16 mm) are advanced across the strictured pylorus and inflated sequentially. Procedural variables that have not been standardized or studied include the duration of insufflation, frequency of dilatation, and size of balloons. The main morbidity of this procedure is perforation requiring emergency operation, with reported rates ranging from 0% to 6%. Performing repeated endoscopic balloon dilatations may risk further scarring of the duodenum, which may lead to a complicated duodenal stump closure if subsequent resection is required. Finally, it must be recognized that this treatment may delay the diagnosis of an obstructing cancer.

## Operative Management

Operative treatment is indicated for most good risk patients who fail conventional medical treatment for obstructing peptic ulcer. Operative treatment is also indicated for patients who have persistent or recurrent symptoms after two or three endoscopic balloon dilatations. Finally, operative treatment is indicated for perforation (endoscopic or spontaneous), massive bleeding, and suspicion of cancer. Intraoperative options for obstructing duodenal ulcer include truncal vagotomy and antrectomy, truncal vagotomy and drainage, or highly selective vagotomy and gastrojejunostomy. The addition of a feeding jejunostomy tube should be considered in most all of these patients and especially for the severely malnourished patients.

The ideal operation for successful treatment of obstructing peptic ulcer must relieve the obstruction, control the ulcer disease, have low morbidity and mortality rates, and produce few late complications. It should also diagnose and treat adequately the occasional patient with an obstructing carcinoma. Truncal vagotomy and antrectomy (TV/A) is the most definitive operation for obstructing peptic ulcer. This operation has the least ulcer recurrence, but as mentioned above, this resective approach might be a less valuable asset in the modern era when elimination of causative factors should minimize the risk of ulcer recurrence perhaps without the need of a major, extirpative procedure. Another potential advantage of TV/A is in the treatment of type 2 (gastric and duodenal) or 3 (prepyloric) gastric ulcers associated with outlet obstruction. Distal gastric resection remains the procedure of choice for gastric ulcer, both because of the cancer risk and because it eliminates the area where recurrent or persistent gastric ulcer may occur. Vagotomy should be performed, because type 2 and type 3 gastric ulcers tend to behave clinically like duodenal ulcers, and acid hypersecretion is thought to be more important in the pathophysiology of these lesions than in the more common, type 1 gastric ulcers.

There are clearly disadvantages to the routine use of TV/A for obstructing peptic ulcer. The operative mortality is about double that of the other (nonextirpative) procedures mentioned above, and the procedure should be avoided in hemodynamically unstable patients and in debilitated or poor risk patients. Also, after TV/A, a substantial number of patients (5–10%) may develop postgastrectomy problems, e.g. dumping, postvagotomy diarrhea, delayed gastric emptying, and afferent or efferent limb problems. Prior to recommending an elective TV/A, the surgeon should ask his-or herself, "How would this patient look 10 pounds lighter?" If the answer to this question is anything other than "fine," another surgical option should be considered. This consideration is especially pertinent to the asthenic female. Finally, resection should be avoided in patients with extensive inflammation and/or scarring of the proximal duodenum, because a secure anastomosis (Billroth I) or duodenal closure (Billroth II) may be compromised.

Truncal vagotomy and drainage (TV/D) with a gastrojejunostomy is advantageous, because an experienced surgeon can perform this procedure quickly and safely. This operative approach also affords the surgeon the opportunity to biopsy the area of obstruction and can be performed as a minimally invasive or laparoscopic-assisted operation. Finally, in the event that dumping is debilitating, the gastrojejunostomy can be reversed provided there is a patent pyloric channel. The main disadvantages of TV/D are the side effects (10% dumping and/or diarrhea) and a 10% rate of recurrent ulcer. Pyloroplasty should be avoided in patients with obstructing peptic ulcer except for the occasional patient with a discrete juxtapyloric stricture. In most patients with obstructing peptic ulcer, Heinecke-Mikulicz pyloroplasty is difficult or impossible. Jaboulay pyloroplasty has been shown in a small prospective clinical trial to be inferior to resection or gastrojejunostomy. Moreover, because recurrent ulceration after TV/D is a possibility, all types of pyloroplasty may make subsequent distal gastric resection, if necessary, more difficult.

Highly selective vagotomy (also called parietal cell or proximal gastric vagotomy) and gastro-jejunostomy is a good option for many patients requiring operation for obstructing peptic ulcer. It is a low risk procedure that treats both the ulcer diathesis (highly selective vagotomy) and the obstruction (gastrojejunostomy). It can be performed as a laparoscopic-assisted procedure, and the gastrojejunostomy is potentially reversible. Preservation of the vagal innervation to the distal stomach supposedly allows the antral propulsive activity to return to normal once the obstruction is bypassed; this may lead to improved gastric emptying. Marginal ulceration may be more common after this operation than after TV/A or TV/D, but some chronic oral acid suppressive medication can be prescribed easily and safely. Moreover, if causative factors (helicobacter, NSAIDs, smoking) are eliminated, risk of recurrent ulcer should be minimized. If recurrent ulceration develops, a secondary operation (thoracoscopic vagotomy or distal gastrectomy) can be performed in a straightforward manner. The disadvantage of highly selective vagotomy and gastrojejunostomy is the risk of marginal ulceration and the risk of dumping from bypassing the pylorus. There has been one randomized, controlled clinical trial on surgical treatment of obstructing duodenal ulcer. Csendes et al. enrolled 90 patients and compared highly selective vagotomy + gastrojejunostomy, highly selective vagotomy + Jaboulay gastroduodenostomy, and selective vagotomy + antrectomy. Mean follow-up was 98 months. Highly selective vagotomy + gastrojejunostomy and selective vagotomy + antrectomy were found to be better than highly selective vagotomy + Jaboulay gastroduodenostomy in terms of patient symptoms on late follow-up. Based on their findings, the authors recommended highly selective vagotomy + gastrojejunostomy as the treatment of choice for obstructing duodenal ulcers, provided the surgeon has experience performing highly selective vagotomy.

The surgeon treating patients with obstructing peptic ulcer should be ever mindful of the possibility of malignant gastric outlet obstruction. One drawback of the minimally invasive approach to treating obstructing peptic ulcer maybe the increased difficulty in appreciating a mass that would be readily apparent by palpation during an open procedure. The surgeon should not hesitate to convert to open operation if the suspicion for cancer is high. Even if the suspicion of cancer is not high, early open reoperation should be considered in the patient who does poorly after TV/D or HSV/GJ.

## Conclusion

For many patients with obstructing peptic ulcer, endoscopic balloon dilatation combined with medical therapy is a practical, initial approach; however, long-term follow-up data are sparse, and patients often require repeated dilatations. Most good-risk patients with gastric outlet obstruction from chronic peptic ulcer disease are best served ultimately by operation.

A high index of suspicion for carcinoma (the most common cause of gastric outlet obstruction nowadays) must be maintained. Vagotomy and antrectomy, truncal vagotomy and gastrojejunostomy, and highly selective vagotomy and gastrojejunostomy are all reasonable options depending on the circumstances. Resection should be avoided in high-risk patients, those with a chronically thin body habitus, and patients with a difficult duodenum. Highly selective vagotomy (or truncal vagotomy) and gastrojejunostomy is an excellent choice for many patients, and these procedures can often be accomplished with minimally invasive techniques. Highly selective vagotomy has the theoretic advantage of maintaining innervation to the antropyloric muscle and avoiding the occasionally severe postvagotomy syndromes. Diagnosis of an occult cancer may be easier with an open operation. Gastric ulcers are best resected if this can be done safely.

# Selected Readings

Awan A, Johnston DE, Jamal MM (1998) Gastric outlet obstruction with benign endoscopic biopsy should be further explored for malignancy. Gastrointest Endosc 48:497–500

Behrman SW (2005) Management of complicated peptic ulcer disease. Arch Surg 140:201–208

Boylan JJ, Gradzka MI (1999) Long-term results of endo-scopic balloon dilatation for gastric outlet obstruction. Dig Dis Sci 44:1883–1886

Csendes A, Maluenda F, Braghetto I et al. (1993) Prospective randomized study comparing three surgical techniques for the treatment of gastric outlet obstruction secondary to duodenal ulcer. Am J Surg 166:45–49

Gibson JB, Behrman SW, Fabian TC, Britt LG (2000) Gastric outlet obstruction resulting from peptic ulcer disease requiring surgical intervention is infrequently associated with *Helicobacter pylori* infection. J Am Coll Surg 191:32–37

Guzzo JL, Duncan M, Bass BL et al. (2005) Severe and refractory peptic ulcer disease: the diagnostic dilemma. Dig Dis Sci 50:1999–2008

Harbison SP, Dempsey DT (1995) Peptic ulcer disease. Curr Prob Surg 42:335–454

Kochhar R, Sethy PK, Nagi B, Wig JD (2004) Endoscopic balloon dilatation of benign gastric outlet obstruction. J Gastroenterol Hepatol 19:418–422

Millat B, Fingerhut A, Borie F (2000) Surgical treatment of complicated peptic ulcers: controlled trials. World J Surg 24:299–306

Perng C-L, Lin H-J, Lo W-C et al. (1996) Characteristics of patients with benign gastric outlet obstruction requiring surgery after endoscopic balloon dilation. Am J Gastroenterol 91:987–990

Zittel TT, Jehle EC, Becker HD (2000) Surgical management of peptic ulcer disease today-indication, technique and outcome. Langenbeck's Arch Surg 385:84–96

# 13
# Peptic Ulcer Disease: Hemorrhage

**John B. Ammori and Michael W. Mulholland**

## Pearls and Pitfalls

- Hemorrhage is the most common complication of peptic ulcer disease (PUD).
- The two most common causes of PUD are: infection with *Helicobacter pylori* and the use of nonsteroidal anti-inflammatory drugs (NSAIDs).
- Approximately 80% of bleeding episodes resolve spontaneously.
- Endoscopy is essential for early diagnosis and treatment.
- Eradication of *H. pylori* reduces rebleeding rates.
- Proton pump inhibitors are warranted after therapeutic endoscopy, when endoscopy is unavailable or delayed, and in patients with hemodynamic instability.
- Rebleeding is best treated endoscopically, except in elderly (>60 years) patients and those with clinically significant comorbid disease.
- Operative intervention is indicated for initial bleeding that cannot be controlled endoscopically, rebleeding in an elderly patient or one with clinically significant comorbidities, and after two rebleeding episodes in other patient populations.
- Ulcer excision is performed for gastric ulcers while duodenal ulcers are managed by direct suture of the ulcer bed.

K.I. Bland et al. (eds.), *Surgery of the Esophagus and Stomach*, DOI: 10.1007/978-1-84996-438-8_13, © Springer-Verlag London Limited 2011

# Introduction

Peptic ulcer disease (PUD) remains a worldwide health concern. The three most common complications of PUD are bleeding, perforation, and obstruction. Peptic ulcer bleeding is the most common complication, occurring in 10–15% of patients during the disease course and is responsible for approximately 40% of deaths resulting from peptic ulcer. Peptic ulcer is the most common cause of upper gastrointestinal (UGI) bleeding, accounting for more than half of UGI bleeding. Bleeding occurs more commonly from ulcers in the duodenum rather than the stomach, often due to posterior erosion into the gastroduodenal artery. With the recognition of the importance of *Helicobacter pylori*, medical treatment of PUD has evolved over the past 20 years. In spite of treatment advances, the incidence of complicated disease has not changed. The number of operations for bleeding has decreased dramatically as endoscopy has become mainstay therapy. Despite these factors, the mortality rate (8–10%) has remained stable as a result of the changing demographics of PUD bleeders to an older patient population with more attendant comorbidities. There has also been a shift in the type of operations performed, with an increase in the use of local procedures combined with eradication of *H. pylori*. An aggressive, but rational approach is crucial for safe diagnosis and management.

# Basic Science

The most common cause of PUD worldwide is *Helicobacter pylori*. The organism is estimated to infect up to 60% of the world's population and leads to peptic ulceration in 6–20% of the infected population. *H. pylori* infestation is associated with 60–70% of gastric ulcers and 90% of duodenal ulcers. For reasons that are not well understood, infection is 15–20% more prevalent in patients with uncomplicated ulceration relative to those with bleeding ulcers.

*H. pylori* is a spiral, gram-negative bacterium first described by Warren and Marshall in 1983. After colonization of the gastric lumen, bacterial and host responses are elicited. *H. pylori* produces urease, an enzyme which hydrolyzes urea to produce ammonia, thereby neutralizing gastric acid to provide an optimal microenvironment for survival. Urease production appears to be critical to the pathogenicity of *H. pylori*, because mutant strains of *H. pylori* without urease activity are unable to produce colonization. The bacterium passes through the mucous layer of the stomach and becomes attached to the gastric epithelium. When attached, *H. pylori* causes direct cellular injury and changes gastric secretory physiology. Infected patients have increased levels of circulating gastrin and decreased somatostatin levels. These endocrine alterations lead to increased basal and maximal acid outputs; acid secretory abnormalities return to normal after bacterial eradication. Interestingly, the bacterium does not colonize the duodenal epithelium at sites of ulceration.

The second most common cause of PUD is the use of non-steroidal anti-inflammatory drugs (NSAIDs). Ulceration occurs by inhibition of prostaglandin production; local prostaglandins normally protect the gastric mucosa by stimulating mucus and bicarbonate production. Approximately 1–4% of chronic NSAID users will develop a peptic ulcer. NSAID use accounts for 25–30% of gastric ulcers and 5–10% of duodenal ulcers. *H. pylori*-positive patients who use NSAIDs have a two-fold increased risk of bleeding compared with *H. pylori*-negative NSAID users.

# Initial Presentation and Assessment

Patients with bleeding peptic ulcers present commonly with hematemesis with or without melena. If the bleeding is massive, hematochezia may occur. Nasogastric lavage yielding blood or "coffee-ground" material confirms an UGI bleed. A negative lavage does not exclude an UGI bleeding occurring in the duodenum distal to a closed pylorus.

Initial assessment must include a medication history to determine the use of NSAIDs, anticoagulants, and anti-platelet agents. Vital signs are obtained to document signs of hypovolemia and shock. Resuscitation begins immediately with the infusion of crystalloid fluids through two large bore (14 or 16 Ga) intravenous lines in the antecubital spaces. Patients are transfused with packed red blood cells if vital signs do not normalize after 2 l of crystalloid or if there is evidence of continuing substantive blood loss. Patients who are unable to protect their airway risk aspiration and should be intubated endotracheally.

After vital signs have stabilized, the patient should undergo an esophagogastroduodenoscopy (EGD) as the diagnostic test of choice. Initial endoscopy should be performed emergently in high-risk patients, such as the elderly and those with major comorbidities, and ideally within 24 h in all patients. Thirty to 90 min prior to EGD, 250 mg of erythromycin may be given intravenously to promote gastric emptying and improve visibility of the gastric mucosa. The diagnostic goals of EGD are to localize the bleeding site and determine the risk for rebleeding. The ulcer can be graded by the Forrest classification (Table 13.1). The risk of recurrent bleeding can be predicted based on ulcer size (>1 cm) as well as the endoscopic appearance of the ulcer bed (Table 13.2). Therapeutic management is dictated by the endoscopic appearance as discussed below.

TABLE 13.1. Forrest classification of Bleeding Peptic Ulcer (Modified from Forrest, 1974).

| Forrest classification | Description |
| --- | --- |
| Ia | Spurting active bleeding |
| Ib | Nonspurting active bleeding |
| IIa | Nonbleeding "visible vessel" |
| IIb | Nonbleeding ulcer with overlying clot |
| IIc | Nonbleeding ulcer with hematin covered base |
| III | Clean ulcer base with no signs of bleeding |

TABLE 13.2. Stigmata of ulcer hemorrhage and risk of recurrent bleeding without endoscopic therapy (Adler et al., 2004. Copyright 2004. With permission from the American Society for Gastrointestinal Endoscopy).

| Stigmata | Risk of recurrent bleeding without therapy |
| --- | --- |
| Active arterial (spurting) bleeding | Approaches 100% |
| Nonbleeding "visible vessel" ("pigmented protuberance") | Up to 50% |
| Nonbleeding adherent clot | 30–35% |
| Ulcer oozing (without other stigmata) | 10–27% |
| Flat spots | <8% |
| Clean-based ulcer | <3% |

Because gastric cancer may present as a bleeding ulcer, multiple biopsies are required of all gastric ulcers. Duodenal ulcers are associated rarely with a malignancy, and therefore biopsies are not mandatory unless indicated by the presence of a mass. All patients should undergo testing for *H. pylori* by rapid urease test, though this test may have reduced sensitivity during an active bleed; specificity, however, approaches 100% even during active bleeding. If the rapid urease test is negative, serologic testing for IgG antibody can be performed, as well as histologic assessment of biopsy material taken from the gastric antrum during endoscopy.

## Treatment and Outcome

EGD is not only the diagnostic test of choice, but also acts as the potential first line therapeutic option. Approximately 80% of peptic ulcer bleeding resolves spontaneously with medical therapy alone. The indications for therapy are based on the endoscopic appearance of the ulcer. Ulcers associated with actively spurting vessels, non-bleeding "visible vessels," or adherent clot should be treated. Endoscopic therapy is not required for lesions with slow oozing and no other stigmata, flat pigmented spots, or clean-based ulcers.

The three major modalities used during endoscopic therapy are injection therapy, thermocoagulation, and mechanical therapy. Injection therapy acts primarily by tamponade due to the volume effect with a secondary pharmacologic effect dependent on the agent used. Epinephrine secondarily causes vasoconstriction; in contrast, ethanol, ethanolamine, and polidocanol are sclerosants that cause direct tissue injury and thrombosis, while thrombin and fibrin provide a hemostatic seal. Thermocoagulation involves the use of a probe positioned on the bleeding site to provide local tamponade followed by application of heat or electrocoagulation to achieve coagulative coaptation. Mechanical methods include endoclip placement or band ligation. Several trials have compared these methods, as well as treatment with combinations of modalities. One prospective, randomized study showed improvements in rebleeding rates, need for operative intervention, and mortality with combination therapy. With injection of 1–2 ml of epinephrine (1:10,000 dilution) and the addition of either thermocoagulation or endoclip placement, initial hemostasis was achieved in 98% of patients.

After successful endoscopic therapy, aggressive medical management is required to prevent recurrent bleeding. All patients with a positive rapid urease test should be treated aggressively with antibiotic therapy to eradicate *H. pylori* with a planned reevaluation in 6 weeks to confirm eradication of the *H. pylori*. A recent meta-analysis demonstrated a rebleeding rate of only 2% after successful eradication of *H. pylori* colonization, a marked and persistent reduction compared with untreated patients. NSAIDs should be withheld during the acute recovery period and indefinitely, if possible. Short-term intravenous proton pump inhibitors (PPIs) are recommended to reduce rebleeding risk for all patients who required endoscopic treatment, particularly in elderly patients with comorbid diseases. Additionally, PPIs should be considered prior to initial endoscopy for patients who present with hemodynamic instability, need for blood transfusions, or delay in endoscopic evaluation. Initiation of PPI therapy should never delay or supersede endoscopy in an actively bleeding patient. H2-receptor antagonists, however, are often ineffective in preventing rebleeding. Maintenance acid suppression therapy is not required after eradication of *H. pylori*. Patients who are NSAID-dependent should be maintained on chronic PPI therapy, as should the small percentage of patients whose ulcer diathesis is unrelated to NSAID use or *H. pylori* infection.

After initial endoscopic hemostasis, 10–25% of patients will rebleed. Gastric ulcers along the lesser curvature and posterior wall duodenal ulcers have the highest risk of rebleeding. Nearly all rebleeding occurs within 48–96 h of the initial intervention. Some surgeons advocate a second-look endoscopy 24 h after initial treatment for possible re-treatment of the high-risk lesions. This approach remains controversial and cannot be recommended as routine. Recurrent bleeding should be treated with aggressive resuscitation and repeat therapeutic endoscopy, which can control approximately 75% of rebleeding episodes with reduced morbidity and no difference in mortality compared with operative therapy. There is, however, a subset of high-risk patients, defined by age >60 years and the presence of major comorbid conditions, who have improved outcomes with early operative intervention rather than a second endoscopic treatment. These patients are not capable of sustaining either the prolonged hypotension or the episodic anemia related to delayed definitive operative control of the bleeding site.

Emergency operative intervention for bleeding peptic ulcers is required in 10–20% of patients hospitalized for UGI bleeding. Operation is indicated for active hemorrhage that is either refractory or inaccessible to initial therapeutic endoscopy. After successful endoscopic control initially, rebleeding is an indication for operative treatment. Elderly patients and those with severe comorbid conditions should undergo operation after the first bleeding recurrence, while most others should be given a chance at a second therapeutic endoscopy; should this second endoscopic treatment fail or the patient rebleed, operative intervention is recommended.

The primary goal of operative therapy for bleeding PUD is stopping the hemorrhage. Bleeding gastric ulcers should be resected, whenever possible. Resection of the ulcer achieves hemostasis, while also providing tissue to examine for gastric cancer. For ulcers located high on the lesser curve of the stomach near the gastroesophageal junction, resection may be difficult. In this situation, there are several options. One option is direct suture ligature of the ulcer base, as well as multiple biopsies to exclude cancer. Other options include resection with gastroplasty closure, or distal gastrectomy extended along the lesser curve to include the ulcer (Pauchet procedure).

For bleeding duodenal ulcers, a Kocher maneuver provides best access to the duodenum. Through a lateral (usually longitudinal) duodenotomy, four quadrant intraluminal suture ligatures are placed around the bleeding vessel at the base of the ulcer. Extraluminal ligation of the gastroduodenal artery has been described, but generally is unnecessary unless intraluminal ligation fails. Special care should be taken to avoid the common bile duct, which passes behind the first and second portions of the duodenum. Figure 13.1 demonstrates a treatment algorithm for UGI bleeding caused by PUD.

Prior to the current appreciation and understanding of the role of *H. pylori* and NSAIDs, a secondary goal of operative treatment was reduction of gastric acid output in order to prevent ulcer recurrence. Acid reduction can be achieved by removal of vagal input (vagotomy) with or without the removal of gastrin-producing G cells of the antrum (antrectomy). Several options are available, which include truncal vagotomy and pyloroplasty, highly selective vagotomy (also called parietal cell or proximal gastric vagotomy), and truncal vagotomy and antrectomy. Studies performed prior to the understanding of the importance of *H. pylori* showed that there was no difference in mortality, but a higher rebleeding rate with local hemorrhage control versus local hemorrhage control plus an antiulcer procedure. With effective therapy to eradicate *H. pylori* and

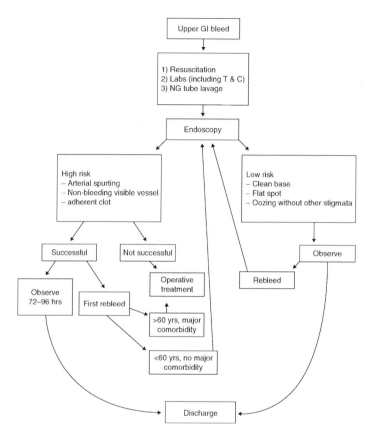

FIGURE 13.1. Algorithm for the treatment of patients with upper gastrointestinal bleeding from peptic ulcer disease (Reprinted from Cowles and Mulholland, 2001. With the permission of Lippincott Williams & Wilkins).

avoidance of NSAIDs, 95% of ulcers are cured. In patients who are NSAID-dependent, chronic PPI therapy will decrease ulcer rates. For these reasons, an acid-reducing operation is indicated only rarely. NSAID-dependent patients who are intolerant of PPI therapy may be candidates for a true anti-ulcer procedure.

# Selected Readings

Adler DG, Leighton JA, Davila RE et al. (2004) ASGE guideline: the role of endoscopy in acute non-variceal upper-GI hemorrhage. Gastrointest Endosc 60:497–504

Calvet X, Vergara M, Brullet E et al. (2004) Addition of a second endoscopic treatment following epinephrine injection improves outcome in high-risk bleeding ulcers. Gastroenterology 126:441–450

Cowles RA, Mulholland MW (2001) Surgical management of peptic ulcer disease in the Helicobacter era-Management of bleeding peptic ulcer. Surg Laparo End Perc Tech 11:2–8

Erstad BL (2001) Proton-pump inhibitors for acute peptic ulcer bleeding. Annals Pharmacol 35:730–740

Feldman RA, Eccersley AJ Hardie JM (1998) Epidemiology of Helicobacter pylori: acquisition, transmission, population prevalence and disease-to-infection ratio. Brit Med Bull 54:39–53

Forrest JAH (1974) Endoscopy in gastrointestinal bleeding. Lancet 304: 394–397

Gisbert JP, Khorrami S, Carballo F et al. (2004) *H. pylori* eradication therapy vs. antisecretory non-eradication therapy (with or without long-term maintenance antisecretory therapy) for the prevention of recurrent bleeding from peptic ulcer. Cochrane Database of Systematic Reviews 2:CD004062

Lau JY, Sung JJ, Lam YH et al. (1999) Endoscopic retreatment compared with surgery in patients with recurrent bleeding after initial endoscopic control of bleeding ulcers. New Engl J Med 340:751–756

# 14
# Gastric Ulcer

Cheong J. Lee and Diane M. Simeone

## Pearls and Pitfalls

- Gastric ulcers comprise 20% of all peptic ulcer disease and can form in the presence of low to normal acid secretion: *Type I* and *IV* Gastric ulcers are not associated with acid hypersecretion, whereas *Types II* and *III* ulcers involve acid hypersecretion.
- All patients with suspected gastric ulcer disease should be evaluated for *H. pylori* infection.
- Endoscopy is the diagnostic modality of choice for evaluating gastric ulcer. Multiple biopsies of an ulcer (at least 7) is required to effectively exclude an underlying neoplasm.
- High suspicion of malignancy should be maintained in older patients with gastric ulcer and those with refractory disease.
- Persistent ulcers after 12 weeks of maximal medical therapy are considered to have refractory disease and require surgical management.
- Choice of operative therapy depends upon the type of gastric ulcer encountered.
- Laparoscopic repair of perforated ulcers have equivalent outcomes when compared with conventional operations.
- Complications of gastric ulcer surgery include: delayed gastric emptying, dumping syndrome, postvagotomy diarrhea, chronic gastroparesis, alkaline reflux gastritis, and afferent or efferent loop syndrome.

K.I. Bland et al. (eds.), *Surgery of the Esophagus and Stomach*, DOI: 10.1007/978-1-84996-438-8_14, © Springer-Verlag London Limited 2011

# Epidemiology and Pathophysiology

Peptic ulcer disease remains a major public health problem, affecting more than 4 million people in the United States. Even with the discovery and elucidation of *Helicobacter pylori*'s role in peptic ulcer formation and subsequent advancement in medical therapy, mortality and complications from peptic ulcer disease still remain substantial as a growing cohort of aging patients with comorbidities seek treatment; ulcer disease is listed as a contributing cause of death in more than 10,000 cases annually. The pathogenesis of peptic ulceration is complex and multifactorial, but often considered an alteration in the balance between acid-peptic secretion and mucosal defense. Luminal secretion of acid is essential to ulcer formation ("no acid – no ulcer"). Unlike duodenal ulcers, gastric ulcers, which comprise about 20% of peptic ulcer disease, may form in the presence of low to normal acid secretion, attesting to the theory that compromised mucosal defense is prerequisite for ulcer formation. Mucosal infection with *Helicobacter pylori* is implicated in the pathogenesis of ulcer formation in most patients. Environmental factors such as ingestion of non steroidal anti-inflammatory drugs (NSAIDS) and cigarette smoking are other important contributors in compromising gastric mucosal defense. A number of rare familial syndromes associated with gastric ulcerations have been described, but there is no clear racial predilection for ulcer development.

# Clinical Presentation and Diagnosis

The classic symptom of peptic ulcer disease is epigastric pain. Patients typically complain of burning, gnawing, or stabbing pain of the upper abdomen that is worse in the morning. Ingestion of food or antacids generally provides relief. Physical exam findings are minimal in uncomplicated cases. A number of patients who are asymptomatic may present with microcytic anemia and guaiac-positive stools. Patients with accompanying anorexia, gastric outlet obstruction, and weight loss should be thoroughly evaluated for the presence of malignancy. The differential diagnosis to consider is broad and includes a wide variety of diseases of the upper gastrointestinal tract, including nonulcerative dyspepsia, gastroesophageal reflux disease, gastric neoplasms, along with inflammatory and neoplastic disease encompassing the pancreas, and cholelithiasis. Less commonly, ulcer pain may be mimicked by mesenteric ischemia or coronary artery disease.

All patients with suspected gastric ulcer disease should be evaluated for *H. pylori* infection. Simple noninvasive diagnostic tests such as serologic antibody testing, urea breath testing, and stool antigen screening are available for initial assessment. In younger patients with mild or intermittent symptoms without systemic symptoms or ulcer complications, treatment following non-invasive testing is appropriate, while in older patients, further diagnostic measures should be taken.

Presently, endoscopy has become the preferred method of evaluating patients with suspected ulcer disease. In a controlled trial comparing endoscopy with barium contrast examination, endoscopy was both more sensitive (92% vs 54%) and more specific (100% vs 91%) in its diagnosis. Endoscopy also allows for biopsy of the mucosa, which is critical in confirming the diagnosis, as well as to rule out neoplasm. Obtaining at least seven biopsy samples of the ulcer is required to effectively exclude an underlying neoplasm.

Traditionally, gastric ulcer has been categorized based upon its anatomic location (Fig. 14.1). *Type I* ulcers are most common (50%) and occur in the body of the stomach along the lesser curvature at the incisura. Patients with *Type I* ulcers have low to normal acid secretion. *Type II* gastric ulcers (25%) also occur along the lesser curvature, but are associated with a duodenal ulcer component. *Type II* ulcers are associated with acid hypersecretion, as are *Type III* ulcers (20%), which are located in the prepyloric region. *Type IV* ulcers (<10%) occur high along the lesser curvature of the stomach

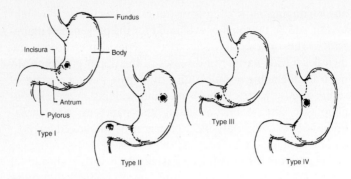

FIGURE 14.1. Types of gastric ulcers.

near the gastroesophageal junction. *Type IV* ulcers are associated with low to normal acid secretion (see Table 14.1).

## Medical Therapy

Once diagnosis has been confirmed and malignancy ruled out, the goal of the therapy is directed towards elimination of the inciting causes of ulcer formation, eradication of *H. pylori* and reduction of acid secretion. Patients should be questioned regarding the use of ulcerogenic agents, namely non steroidal anti-inflammatory agents or steroids, which should be discontinued or weaned as much as possible. In the absence of treatment, spontaneous healing of *H. pylori* infected ulcers occurs in less than 1% of cases. Most widely used treatment regimens include a combination of an antisecretory drug, commonly the H2 receptor antagonist ranitidine or the proton pump inhibitor omeprazole, along with two antibiotics, clarithromycin and amoxicillin or metronidazole. Most series find triple combination antibiotic therapy to be more effective than a single antimicrobial agent, with treatment of patients with triple therapy for 7–14 days resulting in ulcer healing in greater than 90% of patients after 8 weeks on repeat endoscopy. Those with gastric ulcer unrelated to *H. pylori* infection should stop the inciting agent and be placed on antisecretory therapy. In patients that require

TABLE 14.1. Types of gastric ulcers and recommended surgical treatment.

| Gastric ulcer | % incidence | Location | Acid secretion | Recommended surgical management |
|---|---|---|---|---|
| Type I | 50 | Body of the stomach along the lesser curvature | Low | Billroth I or II |
| Type II | 25 | Body of the stomach along the lesser curvature with duodenal ulcer component | High | Billroth I or II + vagotomy |
| Type III | 20 | Prepyloric region | High | Billroth I or II + vagotomy |
| Type IV | <10 | High along the lesser curvature of the stomach near the gastroesophageal junction | Low | Csendes' gastrectomy or Pauchet + Billroth I |

long-term NSAID or steroid therapy, elective surgery may be considered in management of their ulcer disease. All patients with a documented gastric ulcer should undergo repeat endoscopy 8–12 weeks after therapy to assess healing. If an ulcer has failed to completely heal after 12 weeks of continuous medical therapy or if the patient has more than one recurrence, then the patient is considered to have intractable disease. The differential diagnosis of a non-healing ulcer includes persistent *H. pylori* infection, Zollinger-Ellison syndrome, NSAID abuse, mesenteric ischemia, and microscopic malignancy. In the presence of a non-healing gastric ulcer, repeat endoscopy with multiple biopsies is recommended to re-evaluate the gastric mucosa for persistent *H. pylori* infection or an occult malignancy. Zollinger-Ellison syndrome should be excluded by examining the patient's basal serum gastrin levels or by performing a secretion stimulation test. Once measures have been taken to rule out occult, treatable causes of intractability, elective surgery can be planned.

## Surgical Therapy: Elective

Surgical intervention for ulcer disease is reserved for patients who have failed or cannot comply with medical therapy or for those that present with complications. Generally, ulcers that have failed maximal medical therapy for 12 weeks or the inability to rule out an occult malignancy are criteria for elective surgical intervention. For *Type I* gastric ulcers, a distal gastrectomy with Billroth I or II (Fig. 14.2) reconstruction is recommended for most patients, since this approach removes both the ulcer and the diseased antrum. Resection of the diseased segment also allows for more thorough evaluation of a potential underlying malignancy. With antrectomy and reconstruction, acid secretory potential is reduced and gastric drainage is accelerated. Low recurrence rates (0–5%) and excellent symptomatic relief are usually achieved. The operative mortality has been reported to range anywhere from 0% to 6%. Since *Type I* gastric ulcers are rarely associated with acid hypersecretion, the addition of a vagotomy is felt to be unnecessary. This is supported by results from a large series

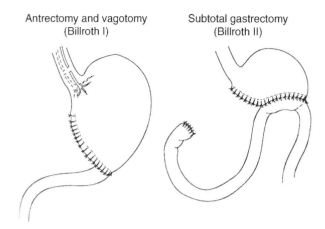

Antrectomy and vagotomy
(Billroth I)

Subtotal gastrectomy
(Billroth II)

FIGURE 14.2.  Billroth I and Billroth II reconstruction (Reprinted from Doherty, 2006. With permission of the McGraw-Hill Companies).

from the Cleveland Clinic reporting on 349 cases of gastric ulcer evaluated from 1950 to 1979. The study found equivalent ulcer recurrence rates following gastric resection for *Type I* gastric ulcer either with or without vagotomy.

Since *Type II* and *III* ulcers are associated with excessive acid secretion, the operative approach includes ulcer excision along with vagotomy. *Type II* gastric ulcers occur synchronously with scarring or ulceration in the duodenum or pyloric channel. They tend to be large, deep ulcers, with poorly defined margins. A truncal vagotomy and antrectomy with Billroth I reconstruction is the preferred surgical option and accomplishes both goals of ulcer excision and decreasing acid secretion. Recurrence rates are less than 5% with an operative mortality rate of about 1%. *Type III* ulcers, which are prepyloric, can also be managed with an antrectomy and vagotomy with Billroth I reconstruction. A Billroth II reconstruction with creation of a gastrojejunostomy can be performed in either *Type II* or *Type III* ulcers if the more physiologic Billroth I reconstruction becomes technically challenging, such as in cases of excessive scarring or inflammation of the duodenum. Highly selective vagotomy is also an option, but has been associated with poor results for both *Type II* and *Type III* ulcers, with ulcer recurrence rates ranging from 16% to 44% in several series.

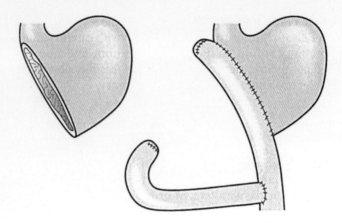

FIGURE 14.3. Csendes' procedure, used to treat gastric ulcers close to the gastroesophageal junction (Reprinted from Csendes et al., 1978, copyright 1978. With permission from Excerpta Medica, Inc).

*Type IV* gastric ulcers are uncommon and may be technically challenging due to their anatomic location high along the lesser curvature, close to the gastroesophageal junction. Ulcer size, distance from the gastroesophageal junction, and surrounding inflammation are important determinants of technical approach. Like *Type I* ulcers, *Type IV* ulcers are not associated with acid hypersecretion and a vagotomy is not necessary. Ulcers that are 2–5 cm from the cardia can be managed with a distal gastrectomy, which is extended along the lesser curvature to include the ulcer (the Pauchet procedure) and a Billroth I reconstruction. For ulcers high up near the gastroesophageal junction, a subtotal gastrectomy with a Roux-en-Y jejunal reconstruction (Csendes' procedure) may have to be undertaken (Fig. 14.3).

## Surgical Therapy: Emergent

Bleeding, perforation, and obstruction are the principal complications of gastric ulcer disease. Because patients with complications from gastric ulcer tend to be elderly and have comorbidities, operation in the emergent setting is associated with high overall mortality, ranging from 10% to 40%. In patients who have bleeding gastric ulcers, indications for emergent operative intervention include: (1) hemodynamic instability despite vigorous resuscitation (>3 unit transfusion), (2) failure of endoscopic techniques to arrest hemorrhage, and (3) recurrent hemorrhage after initial stabilization with up to two attempts at obtaining endoscopic hemostasis. Other relative indications for surgery include rare blood type or difficult crossmatch, refusal of transfusion, shock on presentation, and bleeding chronic gastric ulcer. In hemodynamically unstable patients, vessel ligation with oversewing or excision of the ulcer should be expeditiously performed. If unknown, *H. pylori* status can be determined with mucosal biopsy and rapid urease test. Excision alone, however, is associated with rebleeding in as many as 20% of patients.

In hemodynamically stable patients, a more definitive approach is undertaken with distal gastrectomy and Billroth I or II reconstruction. Bilateral truncal vagotomy is also performed to address acid hypersecretion in patients with *Type II* and *III* ulcers. Patients who undergo truncal or parietal cell vagotomy in this setting have higher ulcer recurrence rates postoperatively, and their use in the urgent or emergent setting is not recommended. With bleeding *Type IV* ulcers, an antrectomy with extension to include the ulcer is preferred. If, however, this approach becomes technically challenging, an alternative approach is to identify and ligate the left gastric artery and to biopsy and oversew the ulcer through a high anterior gastrotomy.

In patients with a perforated gastric ulcer, hemodynamic stability and medical comorbidities become important factors in surgical decision making. The preferred approach to a patient with a perforated ulcer is definitive antrectomy to include the ulcer and, if indicated, a vagotomy. If the patient is at an unacceptably high risk because of advanced age, comorbid disease, intraoperative instability, or severe peritoneal soilage, omental plication of the perforation with biopsy can be performed. In selected patients with a sealed perforation, nasogastric suction, broad spectrum antibiotics, and supportive therapy can be considered. For patients presenting with perforation as their first presentation of gastric ulcer disease with untreated *H. pylori* infection, non-resectional surgical therapy is a reasonable option with medical treatment of *H. pylori* postoperatively. If *H. pylori* is adequately treated, these select patients will have low ulcer recurrence rates. In this cohort of patients, repeat endoscopy should be performed at about 6 weeks postoperatively to gauge appropriate ulcer healing. Any stable patient with a long standing ulcer history should undergo definitive ulcer surgery with an antrectomy and Billroth I or II reconstruction if they develop a perforation. Likewise, in patients with medication induced gastric ulcers that present with perforation, and those medications are essential, definitive anti-ulcer surgery should be planned.

Gastric outlet obstruction is typically a complication of *Type II* and *III* ulcers. Chronic scarring of the duodenum or acute inflammation and subsequent edema is typically the underlying cause. After correction of fluid and electrolyte abnormalities, operation is generally indicated if obstruction fails to resolve after 72 h with antisecretory therapy and naso-gastric tube decompression. In some cases, endoscopic dilatation has been performed successfully; however, the long-term patency rates are not as good as surgical treatment of gastric outlet obstruction. For those patients who undergo surgical intervention, the procedure of choice is an antrectomy with Billroth I or II reconstruction. Placement of a feeding jejunostomy tube at the time of surgery is usually recommended to improve the patient's nutritional status and because the chronic gastric outlet obstruction predisposes delayed postoperative gastric emptying.

## Laparoscopic Surgery

In recent years, laparoscopic surgical approaches have gained popularity for the management of peptic ulcer disease. Several series in the literature demonstrate that a laparoscopic approach is a viable option for perforated peptic ulcer, with outcomes comparable to open surgery. There is growing evidence from these series that laparoscopy is associated with less postoperative pain, reduced pulmonary complications, a shorter postoperative hospital stay, and earlier return to normal daily activities than the conventional open repair. Most of these studies have focused on omental repair of perforated duodenal or juxtapyloric ulcers, and limited evidence exists with regards to repair of other types of perforated gastric ulcers. A laparoscopic approach to operative management of refractory gastric ulcers and gastric ulcers complicated by bleeding and gastric outlet obstruction is feasible, but has not been well-studied.

## Postoperative Management and Potential Complications

In the postoperative period, low continuous nasogastric suction is continued until the patient has evidence of resolving ileus. The patient is supported with intravenous fluids or parenteral nutrition, if indicated, until they are able to maintain oral intake. Patients with prolonged gastric ileus may require enteric feedings through a feeding tube. A naso-enteric feeding access or a feeding jejunostomy can be established at the time of the operation if prolonged ileus is anticipated. Antibiotic use should be limited to perioperative use unless the patient had peritonitis and contamination from a perforated ulcer, in which case, antibiotic use should be continued postoperatively until the patient has resolution of fever and leukocytosis.

Early complications from gastric ulcer surgery are numerous, including superficial and deep infection, bleeding, delayed gastric emptying, and anastomotic leak. In patients who undergo emergent surgical intervention, postoperative complications may develop related to the patients' preexisting comorbidities such as cardiac and respiratory disease. Late sequelae of gastrectomy are thought to be due more in part to the complications associated with vagotomy rather than gastric resection itself, however, have been referred to collectively as the postgastrectomy syndromes. Most patients note a change in their digestive habits postoperatively, and about 20% are significantly affected. Most patients adapt over time with 5% of patients developing lifelong symptoms and 1% of patients severely debilitated by these symptoms. The late complications of gastric ulcer surgery include delayed gastric emptying, dumping syndrome, post vagotomy diarrhea, chronic gastroparesis, alkaline reflux gastritis, and afferent or efferent loop syndrome.

Postvagotomy diarrhea develops in approximately 30% of patients after truncal vagotomy. The condition may be related to the rapid passage of unconjugated bile salts from the denervated biliary tree into the colon, where they stimulate secretion. In most cases, it is self limiting. In persistent cases, cholestyramine administration has been shown to be beneficial.

Dumping syndrome occurs in about 20% of patients after gastrectomy or vagotomy and drainage procedures. Patients experience postprandial gastrointestinal discomfort, which may include nausea, vomiting, diarrhea, and cramps, with vasomotor symptoms such as diaphoresis, palpitations, and flushing. Although the pathogenesis is incompletely understood, the syndrome is frequently attributed to the rapid emptying of hyperosmolar food, particularly carbohydrates, into the small bowel. This causes rapid intraluminal fluid shifts due to the osmotic gradient and may be confounded by the release of one or more vasoactive hormones, such as serotonin and vasoactive intestinal polypeptide. Patients may complain of the same constellation of symptoms hours after eating, called late dumping. This is secondary to hypoglycemia from a postprandial insulin peak and can be managed with carbohydrate ingestion. Most patients with early dumping can be treated conservatively by initiating the dietary changes of frequent small meals that are high in protein and fat and low in carbohydrates. Administration of octreotide has been shown to help in some instances. The rare patient with intractable symptoms may be considered for operative therapy with the goal of delaying gastric emptying, which is best addressed by

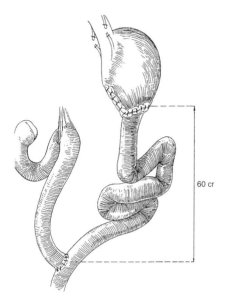

60 cr

FIGURE 14.4. Conversion of an antrectomy with Billroth X reconstruction to a Roux-en-Y reconstruction (Reprinted from Schwartz et al., 1989. With permission of the McGraw-Hill Companies).

converting an antrectomy and Billroth reconstruction to a Roux-En Y reconstruction (Fig. 14.4).

Reflux of bile into the stomach is common after operations that eliminate the pyloric sphincter, but only about 2% of patients that undergo gastric ulcer surgery will experience alkaline reflux gastritis. Alkaline reflux gastritis typically presents with symptoms of postprandial, burning epigastric pain. Although a variety of medical treatments are available, none have been shown to be particularly effective in treating this problem. Surgical revision to a Roux-En Y reconstruction may be necessary to effectively treat this problem, if severe.

Afferent and efferent loop syndromes may develop after Billroth II reconstruction or gastroenterostomy. Patients will complain of postprandial epigastric pain and vomiting in both cases; however, only efferent loop syndrome will present with bilious vomiting. Both are related to mechanical obstruction of the limbs by kinking, anastomotic narrowing, or adhesions. In afferent loop syndrome, the detection of a distended afferent loop on CT is diagnostic. In this setting, operative intervention with a Roux-En Y reconstruction is appropriate.

## Selected Readings

Ashley SW, Evoy D, Daly JM (1999) Stomach In: Schwartz SS, Csendes A, Lazo M, Braghetto I (1978) A surgical technic for (ed) Principles of surgery, 7th edn. McGraw-Hill, New high (cardial or juxtacardial) benign chronic gastric ulcer. York, p 1181 Am J Surg 135:857–858

Doherty GM (2006) Gastric ulcer. In: Doherty GM, Way LW (eds) Current surgical diagnosis and treatment. 12th edn. McGraw-Hill, New York, p 517

Dooley CP, Larson AW, Stace NH et al. (1984) Double-contrast barium meal and upper gastrointestinal endoscopy. A comparative study. Ann Intern Med 101:538–545

Eagon JC, Miedema BW, Kelly KA (1992) Postgastrectomy syndromes. Surg Clin North Am 72:445

Lickstein LH, Matthews JB (1997) Elective surgical management of peptic ulcer disease. Probl Gen Surg 14:37

McDonald MP, Broughan TA, Hermann RE et al. (1996) Operations for gastric ulcer: a long term study. Am Surg 62:673

Ng EK, Lam YH, Sung JJ et al. (2000) Eradication of *Helicobacter pylori* prevents recurrence of ulcer after simple closure of duodenal ulcer perforation: randomized controlled trial. Ann Surg 231:153–158

Schwartz SS, Rodney M et al. (1989) Maingot's abdominal operations, 9th edn. McGraw-Hill/Appleton & Lange, New York, p 716

Siu WT, Leong H, Law BK et al. (2002) Laparoscopic repair for perforated peptic ulcer: a randomized controlled trial. Ann Surg 235:313–319

# 15

# Postgastrectomy and Postvagotomy Syndromes

**Italo Braghetto**

## Pearls and Pitfalls

- Do not submit patients to gastric surgery without a comprehensive, careful evaluation.
- Any operation on the stomach alters normal digestive physiology and can cause symptoms and late sequelae.
- In the past, vagotomy and Billroth I or II gastric resections were used frequently for peptic ulcer disease or gastric cancer and were associated with some element of post gastrectomy/vagotomy syndrome in 25% of patients. These symptoms (diarrhea, early satiety, gastric stasis) were mild, self-limited, and only rarely needed operative treatment.
- Currently, the post-gastrectomy syndromes are rare, because peptic ulcer disease is treated medically.
- For severe, post-gastrectomy gastroparesis, near total gastrectomy with Roux-en-Y reconstruction can be used with successful results in highly selected patients.
- Post-vagotomy diarrhea must be treated with medical and dietary measures; no operative treatment has proven effective.
- Currently, minimally invasive operative procedures for gastric pathology obtain the best functional results.

Operations on the stomach that impair normal gastric and pyloric functions may alter gastrointestinal physiology markedly; collectively, this group of disorders is termed

K.I. Bland et al. (eds.), *Surgery of the Esophagus and Stomach*, DOI: 10.1007/978-1-84996-438-8_15,
© Springer-Verlag London Limited 2011

"postgastrectomy syndromes." Because the postgastrectomy disorders maybe due to varying causes leading to either rapid or delayed gastric emptying and intestinal transit, it is important to differentiate these disorders by careful diagnostic studies, starting by taking a careful history from the patient.

Over the last 50 years, especially before recognizing the importance of *Helicobacter pylori* in the late 1980s/early 1990s, many acid-reducing operations were performed for peptic ulcer disease and gastric cancer. About 25% of these patients developed to some degree symptoms of one or more postvagotomy/post-gastrectomy syndromes. We accumulated considerable experience with managing these disorders, but because only about 1% of patients were permanently disabled, few of these patients required remedial operations. In the last 2 decades, these complications have decreased in incidence and importance due in large part to the changes in the management and operative therapy for peptic ulcer disease; in fact, after 1995, very few elective operations for peptic ulcer have been performed as Stabile and Passaro predicted some years before. Similarly, gastric cancer appears also to be decreasing in many Western countries.

Interestingly, operations for emergencies due mainly to perforation of peptic ulcer disease have remained almost constant, and currently the operative treatment for this disorder can be performed in a conservative way by laparoscopy and omental patch; need for gastrectomy and/or vagotomy is deemed unusual. In similar fashion, elective operations for peptic ulcer disease have declined markedly and nearly disappeared over the last 30 years. This trend preceded the introduction of effective acid-suppressive medications such asH2-receptor antagonists; these drugs, and the more recently developed proton pump inhibitors combined with antibiotic eradication of *Helicobacter pylori* have eliminated effectively the need for elective operative therapy of duodenal ulcer disease. What a remarkable change since the 1960s and 1970s!

Currently, most gastric surgery is performed for malignant diseases and morbid obesity. Advances in perioperative care as well as in operative techniques have decreased the mortality rate after total gastrectomy to less than 2%. Five-year survival after curative resection for gastric neoplasms is in the range of 30–40%, depending obviously on the type, stage, and extent of disease. With the current interest in performing minimally invasive and less aggressive procedures utilizing new technologies, better functional results have led to fewer "post-gastrectomy cripples." In addition, the classic Billroth I or II gastrectomies combined with truncal vagotomy often employed for operative treatment of peptic ulcer disease and for distal gastric cancer have been abandoned in favor of a Roux-en-Y reconstruction of gastrointestinal continuity due to the occurrence of related post-gastrectomy, bile reflux syndromes ("alkaline gastritis," "biliary gastritis," and reflux esophagitis).

Therefore, some of the post-gastrectomy/post-vagotomy syndromes are less common now than over the last 50 years. The physiologic consequences of loss of the stomach, as well as problems related to the method of restoration of gastrointestinal continuity, need to be understood, recognized, diagnosed, and treated if necessary according to the following alterations in gastrointestinal function: abnormal gastric emptying and intestinal transit, disturbed nutritional intake, and abnormal assimilation of ingested nutrients (digestion and absorption). Symptoms can vary considerably and may depend on individual susceptibility, co-morbidities present prior to operation, and the specific type of operative procedures performed. In addition to pathophysiologic changes in gastrointestinal function related to gastrectomy, vagotomy, and methods of reconstruction, it is necessary also to differentiate early or chronic complications due to technical mistakes from the expected physiologic changes of the gastric operation. Afferent loop syndrome, efferent loop syndromes due mesenteric hernias, and mechanical obstructions secondary to adhesive, fibrotic strictures or kinking of the jejunal loop occur not infrequently, can masquerade as post-gastrectomy syndromes, and will respond well to operative correction.

This chapter will review the different postgastrectomy/post-vagotomy syndromes based on the international literature.

# Dumping Syndrome

Dumping has been classified into early and late forms based on the timing of the onset of symptoms after a meal. In patients with early dumping, symptoms start typically 10–30 min after ingestion of a meal. These patients generally have a mixture of gastrointestinal and vasomotor complaints. In contrast, the symptoms in patients with late dumping are primarily vasomotor and occur 2–3 h postprandial. Few patients have both early and late dumping symptoms. The incidence and severity of dumping varies greatly after the various types of gastric surgery. After proximal gastric vagotomy, dumping is quite unusual (<1%); in contrast, after truncal or selective vagotomy with destruction of the pylorus (pyloroplasty, gastroenterostomy, and antrectomy), about 20–30% of patients develop at least some bothersome symptoms, while about 5% have more severe symptoms that can be very severe in about 1%. Vagotomy of the proximal stomach plays a key role in dumping, because antrectomy alone (without vagotomy) and either a Billroth I or Billroth II reconstruction is complicated by dumping in only about 10% of patients. There is some evidence to suggest that clinically important dumping, even after vagotomy, is less common after Roux-en-Y drainage/reconstruction.

**Diagnosis:** Dumping is a clinical diagnosis that depends on the presence of typical symptoms. Abdominal pain is usually absent, but if present, an upper gastrointestinal contrast study and/or upper endoscopy should be performed to exclude stomal obstruction, afferent loop syndrome, or recurrent ulcer as a cause of postprandial pain. In most patients, any further evaluation is usually unnecessary, although a gastric-emptying study can be performed to document rapid gastric emptying. Currently, gastric emptying is assessed by radionuclide markers, including both liquid and solid components of a meal.

The Visick classification can be used to characterize the severity of symptoms after gastric operations and the success of treatment. Visick grade I is no symptoms, Visick II is mild to moderate symptoms not requiring treatment, Visick III is moderate to severe symptoms requiring medical treatment, while Visick IV involves very severe or persistent symptoms affecting quality of life markedly and requiring intense medical management and/or reoperation. Both motor and hormonal mechanisms are involved in the pathophysiology of dumping (Fig. 15.1).

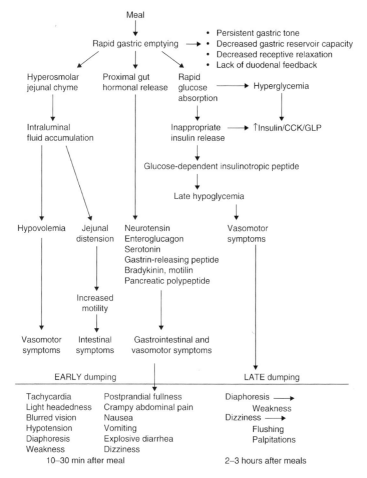

FIGURE 15.1. Pathophysiology of dumping syndrome.

**Treatment:** The treatment of dumping syndrome is largely, in fact almost exclusively, dietary. Based on the known pathophysiologic changes, a diet low in carbohydrate content, "the dry diet routine," and eating small, frequent meals is the first line of treatment in these patients.

Recently, octreotide acetate, a long-acting somatostatin analogue, has been used in treating severe dumping symptoms. Successful resolution of symptoms is unusual, but can be dramatic in up to 20% of patients. Operative treatment is indicated only rarely, because symptomatic relief is usually obtained with medical therapy; moreover, symptoms rarely persist for more than 1 year after the gastric operations.

Many different remedial operations for dumping syndrome have been designed to slow gastric emptying. After vagotomy and pyloroplasty, attempts to reconstruct the pylorus may prove effective. For patients with previous Billroth I or II gastrectomy, Roux-en-Y conversion is the simplest and most effective operation. For patients who have undergone Roux-en-Y gastrojejunostomy, construction of a 10 cm, antiperistaltic jejunal segment within the Roux limb (Christeas' operation) has been suggested; however, although several groups have presented their experience with operative treatment of severe dumping syndrome, the success after these procedures has been disappointing and inconsistent.

## Postvagotomy Diarrhea

Most all types of gastric surgery may result in diarrhea postoperatively, but the incidence of diarrhea is higher in patients who have undergone vagotomy. Truncal vagotomy has the highest incidence of around 20%, whereas the incidence after selective or highly selective vagotomy(which preserves vagal innervation to the small bowel) are 6% and 4%, respectively. Despite its presence, the diarrhea is truly debilitating and only in a small fraction of these patients. Severe symptoms are characterized by frequent watery stools, occasionally explosive, often nocturnal, and not always associated with ingestion of a meal. Occasionally, the diarrhea can occur immediately after a meal concomitant with dumping symptoms. The initial diagnostic approach should include fecal white blood cell count, stool culture, and fecal titers for *Clostridium difficile*. For patients with persistent diarrhea, further studies should be performed to exclude steatorrhea, partial intestinal obstruction, and inflammatory bowel diseases, including fecal-fat studies, upper GI contrast series with small bowel follow-through, and either colonoscopy or barium enema.

Several etiologies for post-vagotomy diarrhea have been proposed, but the exact pathogenesis of this syndrome remains unclear. Gastric stasis leading to bacterial overgrowth, enteritis with malabsorption, changes in small bowel epithelial enzymatic content, decreases in mesenteric blood flow, and denervation of the extrahepatic biliary tree and small intestine leading to rapid transit of unconjugated bile salts into the colon where they inhibit water absorption have also been suggested, but solid experimental work has failed to support any of these theories. Most work suggests that the diarrhea is related to rapid intestinal transit without a true malabsorption.

**Treatment:** Dietary measures that can be effective include a decrease in the intake of both fluid and lactose-containing foods. Antidiarrheal agents, such as diphenoxylate with atropine or loperamide, the bile salt exchange resin cholestyramine, or a trial of octreotide may also be useful. Operative therapy is recommended rarely, because the vast majority of patients with diarrhea early after vagotomy improve with time or dietary changes alone. In our experience, 50% of patients with diarrhea after vagotomy present with mild diarrhea, 40% with more moderate diarrhea, and less than 5% present with daily or incapacitating severe diarrhea. Greater than 90% improve with only dietary modifications and/or medical treatment.

There is, however, the small sub-group of patients with refractive postvagotomy diarrhea. Despite the observation that these patients are miserable, the concept of operative intervention should be approached with caution. Results with one or two, 10 cm anti-peristaltic jejunal interposition(s) are very controversial. In the 1980s, several authors presented successful outcomes claiming that their patients experienced relief from diarrhea; however, several required reoperation for pain or obstruction. Most experts avoid this operation currently. Another procedure reported for treatment of intractable postvagotomy diarrhea is the onlay-reversed-ileal graft designed to create a passive, nonpropulsive segment, thereby slowing small bowel transit; however, the experience in humans is quite limited. Others have attempted to slow transit (and gastric emptying) by conversion to Roux-en-Y gastric emptying but again with infrequent and inconsistent results. Unfortunately, no good treatment exists for these patients.

## Alkaline reflux gastritis (biliary gastritis, biliary gastroesophageal reflux)

Enterogastric reflux is common after Billroth II gastrojejunostomy, but it also occurs after simple gastrojejunostomy, Billroth I anastomosis, or pyloroplasty. Nevertheless, true, symptomatic bile reflux gastritis is quite uncommon, in part, because many surgeons currently prefer Roux-en-Y gastrojejunostomy for reestablishment of gastrointestinal transit after gastrectomy and because gastrectomies are less common today. Which component of the refluxed enteric fluid is the injurious one is not clear, but bile salts are the likely candidate. Interestingly, the severity of the reflux or the severity of the histologic "gastritis" does not correlate with the presence or severity of symptoms. In addition, delayed clearance of bile is also thought to be important in the pathogenesis of this syndrome, and the clinician must be careful not to confuse post-vagotomy gastroparesis with bile reflux gastritis.

**Clinical Presentation:** The symptoms of bile reflux gastritis, although quite rare, are also characteristic. The primary symptom is a characteristic pain. Unlike peptic ulcer pain that is relieved by eating, or gastric ulcer pain that is exaggerated by eating, the pain of bile reflux gastritis is a constant epigastric pain. Bilious vomiting may occur, but the primary symptom is pain.

**Diagnosis:** Endoscopic examination with gastric mucosal biopsy and examination of the gastric anastomosis should be performed to help confirm the diagnosis but also to exclude other diagnoses such as afferent loop syndrome, one of the principal differential diagnoses in patients with bilious vomiting. The endoscopist will see bile pooling within the stomach and often an acutely inflamed, even ulcerated, mucosa. Mucosal biopsies will show intestinalization of the gastric glands, inflammation, and, on occasion, hemorrhage and ulceration, although the severity of the symptoms does not correlate with the histologic changes. Indeed, most all patients after a gastrectomy and with Billroth II reconstruction or after pyloroplasty or loop gastrojejunostomy will have some element of bile within the stomach and gastritis of varying severity. Many gastric surgeons recommend evaluation of gastric emptying, because the symptoms and endoscopic findings of post-vagotomy gastroparesis mimic many of those of bile reflux gastritis, and the treatment of such differs markedly. Scintigraphic assessment of the magnitude of reflux can also be obtained by tagging bile with a radioactive marker and determining the percentage of the secreted isotope refluxed into the stomach.

**Treatment:** Unfortunately, attempts at medical treatment are generally ineffective. The operative approach most often effective is diversion of bile away from the stomach. After a previous gastrectomy, this approach is best accomplished by converting gastric drainage to a Roux-en-Y limb of at least 70 cm (not just the classic 40 cm length). Some consideration may be given to a higher gastrectomy to decrease the possibility of future stomal ulceration. The Henley jejunal interposition limb between the gastric remnant and the duodenum has also been used to treat alkaline reflux gastritis, but we have no experience with this procedure. For patients with documented bile reflux gastritis after pyloroplasty alone (or the rare patient after cholecystectomy), the "duodenal switch" procedure can also be used; this procedure involves transaction of the junction of the first and second portion of the duodenum proximal to the entry of bile into the duodenum, oversewing

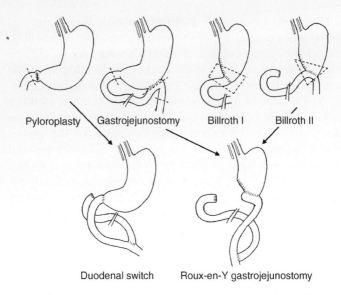

Pyloroplasty    Gastrojejunostomy    Billroth I    Billroth II

Duodenal switch    Roux-en-Y gastrojejunostomy

FIGURE 15.2. Surgical options for treatment of alkaline gastritis.

the distal duodenum, and Roux-en-Y duodeno-jejunostomy (Fig. 15.2).

## Small Gastric-Remnant Syndrome

Early satiety with or without early postprandial vomiting is probably the most common postgastrectomy complaint and occurs often in the first 6 months after gastrectomy. Patients with this syndrome develop a characteristic pattern of early satiety, abdominal fullness, epigastric discomfort or pain, weight loss, nutritional deficiencies, and anemia. In addition, they will often have dumping symptoms. Conservative medical treatment is indicated in most patients and consists of symptomatic relief with antispasmodic agents, dietary counseling, and reassurance, because as the GI tract adapts to this new anatomy, this symptom complex resolves gradually. A very small number of patients develop intractable pain and weight loss despite medical management. In these instances, the clinician should suspect gastroparesis, mechanical obstruction at the anastomosis, or the Roux stasis syndrome (see below). Although several types of surgically constructed complicated pouches have been designed to restore the reservoir function of gastric remnant, none has proven to be successful consistently.

# Roux Stasis Syndrome/Post-Vagotomy Gastroparesis

Patients with the Roux-en-Y esophago-or gastrojejunostomy are at increased risk for delayed emptying secondary to the Roux stasis syndrome. Most investigators believe that this syndrome is secondary to abnormalities in motility of the jejunum distal to the site of transaction used to create the Roux limb which occurs primarily in patients who also have had a vagotomy; this syndrome is very unusual after, for instance, a Roux-en-Y gastric bypass which does not have a vagotomy. The symptoms include epigastric fullness, early satiety, abdominal pain, nausea, and vomiting not of bile but of ingested food. Indeed, these are the same symptoms and the same presentation as gastroparesis. Severe symptoms can lead to malnutrition and progressive weight loss. Gastric bezoars may develop. The spectrum of symptoms occurs to some extent in 10–50% in patients who have had a Roux drainage procedure combined with a vagotomy.

The medical management of this condition is disappointing and consists of dietary modification with smaller, more frequent meals and a more liquid-based diet; several drugs have been used but with highly variable results, including metoclopramide, domperidone (a dopamine antagonist), and cisapride (now no longer available). No completely satisfactory treatment for the Roux-en-Y stasis syndrome is available; attempts at intestinal electrical pacing, while successful in animals, have not worked in humans. When laboratory studies that incriminate the stomach (gastroparesis) as the cause of the stasis rather than the Roux-en-Y limb, near total gastrectomy has been advocated by some authors, and results have been encouraging. Therefore, the Roux-en-Y stasis syndrome should remain a diagnosis of exclusion, and remedial operations to resect the gastric remnant and re-establish the transit with a 40 cm long Roux limb have been proposed. About half the patients will have a reasonable result and be able to maintain their nutrition with oral intake; however, about half will require enteral feeding (distal to the Roux limb) or even total parenteral nutrition.

## Prevention of Post-Vagotomy/ Post-Gastrectomy Problems

Table 15.1 summarizes the most common symptoms after the various types of vagotomy and gastrectomy. Abnormalities discussed above in gastric emptying, intestinal transit, and enterogastric reflux resulting in abnormal digestion and nutrition account for the spectrum of post-vagotomy/post-gastrectomy symptoms and syndromes. Several modifications of the various classic operations have been evaluated in an attempt to prevent these symptoms. Various types of "neogastric pouches" have been constructed using the Roux limb in an attempt to provide a larger reservoir for ingested food; none has been demonstrated to impact consistently on postprandial eating habits, including J-shaped or S-shaped pouches, Omega loops, or interposition jejunal segments between the esophagus and the proximal duodenum. Similarly, the so-called uncut Roux limb has been evaluated in an attempt to prevent the Roux stasis syndrome. This procedure involves creating a loop gastro-or esophago-jejunostomy but stapling across the afferent limb to prevent pancreatobiliary secretions from refluxing into the stomach or esophagus, respectively. Then a side-to-side jejuno-jejunostomy is constructed between the afferent limb just proximal to the occluding staple line and the efferent limb at least 40 cm distal to the gastro- or esophago-jejunostomy. The concept behind this procedure is that by avoiding a complete transaction of the jejunum (to create a

TABLE 15.1. Late symptoms and complications after gastric surgery according to different techniques.

|  | TV + A | SV + A | A alone | HSV |
|---|---|---|---|---|
| Malabsorption | + | ++ | +++ | − |
| Loss of body weight | ++ | ++ | +++ | − |
| Anemia | + | + | ++ | − |
| Dumping | ++ | ++ | +++ | − |
| Diarrhea | +++ | ++ | + | − |
| Cholelithiasis | +++ | − | − | − |
| Alkaline reflux gastritis | ++ | ++ | +++ | − |
| Gastric cancer | ++ | ++ | +++ | − |

TV = total vagotomy; A = antrectomy; SV = selective vagotomy; HSV = highly selective vagotomy.

Roux limb), the motility of the jejunum downstream from the gastro-or esophago-jejunostomy will remain normal; the staple line prevents flow of enteric content but does not interrupt neuromuscular transmission in the wall of the jejunum across the staple line. Small series with this approach are encouraging.

# Selected Readings

Braghetto I (1990) Late complications after surgery of duodenal ulcer. Cuad Chil Cir 34:82–95

Braghetto I, Bosch H, Csendes A (1986) Postoperative diarrhea after surgery for peptic ulcer. Rev Chil Cir 38:124–129

Braghetto I, Csendes A, Parada M, Lazo M (1983) Dumping syndrome. Rev Chil Cir 35:204–210

Carvajal S, Mulhivill SJ (1994) Postgastrectomy syndromes: dumping and diarrhea. Gastroenterol Clin NA 23:261–279

DeMeester TR, Fuchs KH, Ball CS et al. (1987) Experimental and clinical results with proximal and-to-end duodenojejunostomy for pathologic duodenogastric reflux. Ann Surg 206:414–426

Eagon JC, Niedema BW, Kelly KA (1992) Postgastrectomy syndromes. Surg Clin NA 72:445–465

Liedman B, Hugosson I, Lundell L (2001) Treatment of devastating postgastrectomy symptoms. The potential role of jejunal pouch reconstruction. Dig Surg 18:218–221

Mackie CR, Jenkins SA, Hartley MN (1991) Treatment of severe post-vagotomy/postgastrectomy symptoms with the somatostatin analogue octreotide. Br J Surg 78:1338

Schölmerich J (2004) Postgastrectomy syndromes-diagnosis and treatment. Best Proct Res Clin Gastroenterol 18:917–933

# 16
# Bariatric Surgery

**Silas M. Chikunguwo, Stacy A. Brethauer,
and Philip R. Schauer**

## Pearls and Pitfalls

- Obesity affects an estimated 1.7 billion people worldwide.
- Males and females in their twenties with a BMI >40 have 13 year and 8 year shorter life expectancies, respectively, than normal weight persons.
- Accepted criteria for bariatric surgery include a BMI ≥40 or a BMI 35–39 with active weight-related comorbidities and no active substance abuse or uncontrolled psychiatric issues.
- Currently bariatric surgery is the most effective, most durable treatment for weight loss.
- Bariatric surgery resolves the metabolic syndrome, decreases cardiovascular risk (~80%), and resolves or improves glucose intolerance, hypertension, dyslipidemia, sleep apnea, and gastro-esophageal reflux in over 80% of patients.
- Successful weight loss decreases markedly the risk of cardiovascular death and prolongs survival.
- The laparoscopic adjustable gastric band (LAGB) has the lowest morbidity and mortality rate of currently available bariatric procedures; weight loss at 5 years is ~45% of excess body weight.
- Laparoscopic sleeve gastrectomy, while effective as the first stage of a planned two-stage procedure for selected, high risk patients with super morbid obesity, has not yet

K.I. Bland et al. (eds.), *Surgery of the Esophagus and Stomach*, DOI: 10.1007/978-1-84996-438-8_16,
© Springer-Verlag London Limited 2011

been proven to be effective long-term as a primary bariatric procedure.

- Vertical banded gastroplasty is currently performed only rarely because of poor long-term weight loss and multiple complications/side effects.
- Malabsorptive procedures (biliopancreatic diversion and duodenal switch) have excellent and durable weight loss but a higher rate of complications; these procedures are best reserved for selected patients.
- Roux-en-Y gastric bypass is the most common procedure performed in the U.S. and the majority are now performed laparoscopically.
- All bariatric procedures have potential morbidity, both mechanical (operation-specific) and nutritional (malabsorption, micronutrient deficiency, vitamin deficiency: vitaminB12, fat soluble vitamins) and thus, life-long medical follow up is mandatory.

Obesity is defined as the accumulation of excess body fat and is best quantified as body mass index (BMI, weight in kilograms divided by height in meters squared ($kg/m^2$))(Table 16.1). The obesity epidemic in developed countries throughout the world has spawned a tremendous interest in obesity research as well as a dramatic increase in the number of bariatric operations performed each year. Despite current efforts to prevent obesity, the percentage of overweight people in the world continues to rise and now rivals

TABLE 16.1. Classification of obesity.

| Severity | Body mass index ($kg/m^2$) | % Over ideal body weight |
| --- | --- | --- |
| Overweight | 25.0–29.9 | |
| Obesity (Class 1) | 30.0–34.9 | >20% |
| Moderate obesity (Class 2) | 35.0–39.9 | >100% |
| Severe (Morbid) obesity (Class 3) | 40.0–49.9 | |
| Super morbid obesity | >50 | >250% |

the number of underweight people. Severe obesity leads to multiple comorbid conditions (Table 16.2) and decreased life expectancy, and currently, the only effective, durable treatment for this disease is bariatric surgery. Bariatric procedures performed today include malabsorptive procedures (biliopancreatic diversion, duodenal switch), restrictive

TABLE 16.2. Comorbidities associated with obesity.

| | |
|---|---|
| Cardiovascular | Coronary artery disease<br>Hypertension |
| Peripheral vascular | Deep venous thrombosis<br>Pulmonary embolism<br>Thrombophlebitis<br>Venous stasis disease<br>Atherosclerosis Stroke |
| Pulmonary | Asthma<br>Obstructive sleep apnea<br>Obesity hypoventilation syndrome |
| Gastrointestinal | Gastroesophageal reflux<br>Esophagitis |
| Hepatobiliary | Hepatic steatosis<br>Non-alcoholic steatohepatitis (NASH)<br>Cirrhosis<br>Cholelithiasis |
| Neurologic | Migraines<br>Pseudotumor cerebri<br>Depression |
| Malignancy | Colon Breast<br>Endometrium<br>Prostate |
| Musculoskeletal | Degenerative joint disease<br>Gout Carpal tunnel syndrome |
| Gynecologic/urologic | Irregular menstruation<br>Polycystic ovarian syndrome<br>Infertility<br>Stress urinary incontinence<br>Urinary tract infections |
| Metabolic/endocrine | Diabetes (insulin-resistant)<br>Dyslipidemias |

procedures (laparoscopic adjustable gastric banding, vertical banded gastroplasty, sleeve gastrectomy), or procedures that combine these two mechanisms (Roux-en-Y gastric bypass). Each procedure has its unique mechanism of action and associated risks and benefits. As more is learned about the pathophysiology of obesity and the biochemical changes that occur with weight loss after bariatric surgery, new less-invasive procedures will emerge undoubtedly. There is little doubt, though, that the problem of obesity will be present for years to come and that bariatric surgery will play an important role in managing this chronic disease entity.

## Epidemiology

The epidemic of excess weight and obesity affects currently an estimated 1.7 billion people in developed countries throughout the world. As many as 60% of people in the United States are overweight, while the US has the highest prevalence of obesity worldwide (32%). This prevalence has increased dramatically over the last 2 decades, up from 15% in 1980. In the US, the prevalence of extreme obesity (BMI > 40) is 2.8% in men and 6.9% in women. Childhood and adolescent obesity has tripled since 1980 to a prevalence rate of 17%. Overall, the prevalence of obesity continues to increase at an alarming rate on a global scale, particularly in industrialized countries such as the United Kingdom, Australia, Germany, Russia, Columbia, Brazil, Italy, and Austria.

## Costs of Obesity

The costs of obesity are enormous, both in terms of the economic impact of this disease and the medical consequences that result from comorbid conditions. The total cost attributable to obesity in the United States is over $100 billion annually. Worldwide, approximately 2.5 million annual deaths occur due directly to obesity-related comorbidities. The economic costs of obesity include direct medical costs of treating obesity illnesses and indirect costs due to lost work-days, productivity, and future income due to premature death. Epidemiologic studies suggest that, among African Americans, a higher BMI (32 for men, 37 for women) decreases life expectancy. The same study estimated that a Caucasian man in his twenties with a BMI over 45 will have a 22% reduction (13 years) in life expectancy, and a 20 year old Caucasian woman with a BMI of 45 will have 8 years of life lost to obe-sity. For each patient contemplating bariatric surgery, the risks of a bariatric procedure must be weighed against the long-term risks and costs of continued obesity nd worsening comorbidities.

## Surgical Management of Obesity

The dramatic increase in interest in bariatric surgery among surgeons and in the public occurred essentially between 1993 and 2003, when the number of bariatric procedures per-formed annually worldwide increased nearly four-fold to 145,000. Interestingly, membership in bariatric surgery societ-ies has also increased by over 100%. Despite these increasing numbers of operations and the now well-documented suc-cesses of bariatric surgery to date, relatively few eligible patients are pursuing bariatric surgery. Currently, only about 1% of patients eligible for bariatric surgery in the United States have undergone a weight-loss procedure.

Patients with a BMI $\geq$40 kg/m$^2$ or a BMI $\geq$35 kg/m$^2$ with significant obesity-related comorbidities are candidates for bariatric surgery based on the 1991 NIH Consensus Guidelines. Typically, patients between the ages of 18–60 are considered for surgical weight loss. Carefully selected older patients and, increasingly, adolescents as well can benefit from bariatric surgery. Patients seeking bariatric surgery have, throughout their lives, failed multiple attempts at medical weight loss. In addition to meeting the basic criteria for surgery, these patients must also complete a thorough, multi-disciplinary, preoperative evaluation designed to identify and optimally manage comorbid conditions and identify any contraindications to bariatric surgery.

Patients who cannot tolerate general anesthesia due to cardiac, pulmonary, or hepatic insufficiency are obviously not candidates for bariatric surgery. Patients must also demonstrate during their preoperative evaluation that they understand the associated changes in lifestyle required after surgery and are willing to comply with the post-operative diet, vitamin supplementation, and follow-up program. Most importantly, patients must understand that bariatric surgery is only a tool to help them lose weight in conjunction with good choices in food and adoption of an exercise program and not as a rapid solution to a lifelong problem.

Currently, no specific psychologic factors have been identified that predict success or failure reliably after bariatric surgery. Patient selection with regard to psychologic stability is based on the judgment of the psychologist/psychiatrist and the surgeon. Patients with active substance abuse or unstable psychiatric illness, though, are poor candidates for bariatric surgery.

## Outcomes after Bariatric Surgery

**Weight loss:** Bariatric surgery is currently the most effective and durable method to treat severe obesity. Weight loss is most commonly measured as percent of excess weight loss (% EWL). Excess weight is defined as the amount of weight above the patient's ideal body weight (as determined by Metropolitan Life tables).

A meta-analysis by Buchwald and colleagues including over 10,000 patients found an average EWL of 61% for all patients undergoing bariatric surgery. Malabsorptive procedures had the greatest EWL (70%), while gastric banding (including open, non-adjustable gastric bands) had the least EWL (47.5%). The average EWL for Roux-en-Y gastric bypass in this analysis was 62%.

The Swedish Obesity Subjects (SOS) Study is an ongoing, prospective, controlled, matched-pair cohort study comparing surgery with nonsurgical treatment for obesity. The surgically treated patients underwent a variety of procedures, including vertical banded gastroplasty (70%), fixed or adjustable gastric banding (25%), and gastric bypass (5%). The treatment in the nonsurgical group varied widely as well, including intense behavioral therapy to no specific treatment according to the practices of their primary care physicians. Analysis at 10 years (641 surgical and 627 nonsurgical patients) showed that the control group had gained 2% of their original weight, while the surgical group lost 16% of their total body weight. Other studies have demonstrated durable weight loss beyond 15 years for gastric bypass and biliopancreatic diversion.

**Comorbidity reduction:** Bariatric surgery results in a decrease or resolution of many obesity-related comorbid conditions. The Metabolic Syndrome (abdominal obesity, atherogenic dyslipidemia, hypertension, insulin resistance or glucose intolerance, a proinflammatory state, and a prothrombotic state) comprises a constellation of serious cardiovascular risk factors; bariatric surgery improves or leads to resolution of all of these factors in over 80% of patients and decreases the risk for cardiovascular disease. Christou et al. conducted a matched cohort study comparing patients after bariatric surgery with a medically managed cohort and demonstrated an 82% decrease in cardiovascular risk 5years after surgery. Similarly, diabetes also improves dramatically after bariatric surgery. Buchwald's meta-analysis showed that diabetes resolved in 99% of patients after biliopancreatic diversion, 84% after gastric bypass, 72% after gastroplasty, and 48% after gastric banding. About half of morbidly obese patients are hypertensive, and 80%of patients undergoing bariatric surgery will have resolution or improvement in their hypertension and their lipid profile after bariatric surgery.

Sleep apnea, obesity hypoventilation syndrome (Pickwickian Syndrome), and asthma improve or resolve in the majority of patients after massive weight loss.

Gastroesophageal reflux is treated effectively by bariatric procedures. Gastric bypass is particularly effective in treating reflux (70–90% resolution of symptoms) and should be considered strongly instead of a fundoplication for morbidly obese patients with a primary complaint of severe gastroesophageal reflux.

Other comorbidities that improve or resolve after bariatric surgery include non-alcoholic steato-hepatitis, venous stasis disease, lymphedema, pseudotumor cerebri, depression, polycystic ovarian syndrome, and stress urinary incontinence.

**Life expectancy:** Morbid obesity shortens the expected life span, but there is growing evidence that bariatric surgery alters the natural history of this disease. Retrospective, case control studies have demonstrated that 15 year survival is increased by one third for patients undergoing bariatric surgery compared with obese patients who do not have surgery. MacDonald et al. compared retrospectively obese diabetic patients who underwent gastric bypass (n = 154) to a similar group of obese diabetic patients who did not have bariatric surgery (n = 78); at 10 years of follow-up, there was a mortality rate of 9% in the surgical group (including perioperative deaths) but a 28% mortality rate in the nonsurgical group, related to decreased cardiovascular deaths among patients who had gastric bypass. Similarly, in a matched cohort study of 1,035 gastric bypass patients and 6,746 age and sex-matched controls, Christou and colleagues reported a 5-year mortality in the surgical group of about 1% compared with 16% in the medically managed patients (89% relative risk reduction).

**Perioperative mortality:** Mortality rates after bariatric surgery depend on the patient's comorbidities and general risk, the procedure performed, and the surgeon and hospital volume of bariatric cases. The leading cause of death after bariatric surgery is pulmonary embolism (30–40% of deaths) followed by cardiac complications (25%) and anastomotic leaks (20%). The remaining perioperative deaths are due to respiratory, vascular, and hemorrhagic causes.

Restrictive procedures are associated with the lowest perioperative mortality rates (0.1%). A systematic review of the international literature revealed a 0.05% mortality rate after laparoscopic adjustable gastric banding; this procedure is considered the safest bariatric procedure performed today. The mortality rate for gastric bypass (open and laparoscopic) in Buchwald's meta-analysis was 0.5%. Malabsorptive procedures, such as biliopancreatic diversion and duodenal switch, are technically more demanding and are associated with a greater mortality rate than other bariatric procedures (1.1%), but these procedures tend to be performed on larger, higher risk patients.

Advanced age is also associated with higher mortality rates after bariatric surgery. In a review of Medicare patients undergoing bariatric surgery, one study found that patients older than 65 had 4.8% 30-day and 6.9% 90-day mortality rates, which were higher than after bariatric surgery in younger patients.

# Restrictive Procedures

## *Laparoscopic Adjustable Gastric Banding*

The Laparoscopic Adjustable Gastric Band (LAGB) utilizes a restrictive mechanism for weight loss by creating a small gastric pouch just below the gastroesophageal junction (Fig. 16.1a). After opening the pars flacida along the lesser curvature of the stomach, a small window is created in the peritoneum at the base of the right diaphragmatic crus. Another small opening is created just above the angle of His and a blunt instrument is used to create a path for the band behind the cardia of the stomach. After the retrogastric tunnel is created, the band is pulled through and locked in place around the upper stomach just below the gastroesophageal junction. The fundus is then plicated over the band to the gastric wall (not esophagus) above the band using three interrupted sutures, which helps prevent slippage or prolapse anteriorly. The plications should not cover the buckle of the band as this may increase the risk of band erosion. The tubing

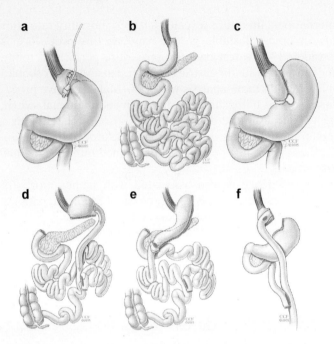

FIGURE 16.1. Restrictive procedures: (a) laparoscopic adjustable gastric band; (b) sleeve gastrectomy; (c) vertical banded gastroplasty. Malabsorptive procedures: (d) biliopancreatic diversion; (e) biliopancreatic diversion with duodenal switch. Combination procedure: (f) Roux-en-Y gastric bypass (Reprinted with the permission of the Cleveland Clinic Foundation).

is attached to the port extracorporeally, and the port is sutured to the anterior rectus fascia. Typically, fluid is not added to the band until 1 month after surgery.

**Advantages:** A major putative advantage of the adjustable band is that the outlet of the gastric pouch can be titrated to weight loss and symptoms. This ability to vary the diameter of the pouch outlet avoids many of the chronic problems (severe reflux, dysphagia, vomiting, and maladaptive eating behaviors) seen with non-adjustable gastric banding. Regular follow-up is essential after the LAGB to achieve the optimal band tightness for each patient. The LAGB is the safest bariatric procedure with a mortality rate of 0.05% and a morbidity rate of 11%. This safety profile makes LAGB an attractive option for many patients and surgeons.

Weight loss after LAGB is more gradual than after gastric bypass, and maximal weight loss is achieved between 2 and 3 years (vs. 12–18 months after gastric bypass). Excess weight loss 3–5 years after LAGB ranges from 40% to 60% and is associated with improvements in most all weight-related comorbidities.

**Complications:** Major perioperative complications such as bleeding, gastric perforation, or thromboembolic events are rare after LAGB and occur in only 1–2% of patients. Late complications that occur after LAGB include device-related problems (port or tubing malfunctions in 5% of patients) or complications such as band slippage (5–15%) or band erosion (1%). Overall, complications require re-operation in 10–15% of patients undergoing LAGB.

## Laparoscopic Sleeve Gastrectomy

Laparoscopic sleeve gastrectomy (LSG) is a relatively new procedure in bariatric surgery. It was introduced initially as a first stage procedure for very high-risk patients (BMI > 60) who ultimately underwent a RYGB. The intent of this first stage is to perform a relatively safe and simple procedure in a patient who cannot tolerate a prolonged anesthetic or who has anatomy that is unfavorable for performing a gastric bypass at that time because of cirrhosis, massive visceral fat, poor exposure due to hepatomegaly, or extensive intra-abdominal adhesions; this remains the primary, accepted indication for this restrictive procedure. But there is growing interest in using the LSG as a primary restrictive procedure. Sleeve gastrectomy has also been used in patients with inflammatory bowel disease, in whom the integrity of an anastomosis is a concern, and in patients with gastric or duodenal polyps in whom performance of a RYGB would make surveillance of this anatomy impossible.

In this procedure, a linear cutting stapler is used to tubularize the lesser curvature by creating a narrow gastric tube along the lesser curvature (Fig. 16.1b). The remaining 75–80% of the gastric body and fundus are removed. Starting approximately 6 cm proximal to the pylorus, the lesser sac is entered through the gastrocolic ligament, and a linear cutting stapler is fired toward the angle of His. A Bougie dilator is used to size the sleeve. We currently use a 34 French Bougie and direct the tip into the pylorus after the initial vertical staple load is fired. Once the Bougie is in place, the stomach is divided adjacent to the dilator up to the Angle of His. The short gastric vessels are then divided and the now resected greater curvature of the stomach remnant is removed.

**Advantages:** This procedure provides a safe and relatively simple procedure for high risk patients or patients with massive hepatomegaly. The procedure has a relatively low complication rate and low mortality rate in the initial series published in very high-risk patients. In these series, patients had impressive initial decreases in weight (50–60% EWL), comorbidities, and anesthetic risk in the first year after LSG prior to the second stage procedure (RYGB). Although LSG has been studied as a primary procedure in lower BMI patients with reported EWL of 50–80% in the first year after surgery and improvement or resolution of many comorbidities, the durability of LSG beyond 1 year, has not been demonstrated. LSG as an effective, durable primary bariatric procedure is thus not yet established or accepted.

**Complications:** LSG appears to be safe and effective in the short term when used as a staged or a primary procedure. Overall, post-operative complications occur in 10–15% of patients and include strictures (most commonly at the gastric incisura), bleeding, and staple line leaks. Complication rates of LSG as a primary procedure are lower than those seen with the high-risk patients who undergo LSG as a staging procedure.

## Vertical Banded Gastroplasty

This procedure (a form of "stomach stapling") involves the creation of a small, vertically oriented proximal gastric pouch, which empties into the main body of the stomach through a calibrated stoma (Fig. 16.1c). The small pouch is created with a linear stapler and can be divided, although historically, the pouch has been created with an undivided staple line (or overlapping staple lines) using a combination of a circular stapler and a linear stapler fired upward from a window to the angle of His. A silastic or polypropylene band is placed around the outlet to provide fixed restriction of the outlet.

Although this procedure was popular in the 1980s and early 1990s, its demonstrated inferior weight loss compared with RYGB and long-term complications such as severe gastroesophageal reflux, nausea and vomiting, intolerance to solid foods, and weight regain in over half of patients who underwent this procedure have discouraged its current use. Many bariatric surgeons are seeing increasing numbers of patients who present for revision to RYGB after failing VBG (severe symptoms or weight regain).

# Malabsorptive Procedures

## Biliopancreatic Diversion and Duodenal Switch

These procedures work by limiting nutrient absorption (Fig. 16.1d). In the biliopancreatic diversion (BPD), a 70% gastrectomy is completed and a long alimentary Roux limb from the proximal ileum is anastomosed to the remaining stomach. The biliopancreatic limb is connected to the alimentary limb about 100 cm from the ileocecal valve to create a short common channel. In the duodenal switch (DS) (Fig. 16.1e), a sleeve gastrectomy is performed and a similar long alimentary Roux limb is anastomosed to the first portion of the duodenum. Again, a short common channel is created by connecting the biliopancreatic limb to the alimentary limb about 100 cm from the ileocecal valve.

**Advantages:** BPD and BPD with duodenal switch (BPD/DS) provide excellent long-term weight loss, with greater than 75% EWL maintained 15 years after the procedure.

Though there is some adaptation of the common channel, the majority of patients are able to consume relatively normal quantities of food yet maintain their weight loss. In addition to weight loss, resolution of comorbid conditions exceed 80% and was superior to most other bariatric procedures in Buchwald's meta-analysis.

**Complications:** Although these procedures offer the best and most durable weight loss of any bariatric procedure performed today, higher complication rates, which include global protein/calorie malnutrition, anemia, micronutrient deficiency, diarrhea, stomal ulceration, metabolic bone disease, and a higher mortality rate, have limited their widespread use. Patients need to be followed closely, especially for fat-soluble vitamin deficiencies.

## Gastric Bypass

The Roux-en-Y gastric bypass (RYGB) (Fig. 16.1f) is the most commonly performed bariatric procedure in the United States (80%) and is performed open or, more commonly, laparoscopically. The primary mechanism of weight loss after gastric bypass is the restrictive component resulting from creating a small gastric pouch and small gastrojejunostomy and possibly initially by setting up a dumping physiology for ingestion of high caloric sweets. A global malabsorption is typically negligible with a standard 75–150 cm alimentary limb. The foregut bypass created with RYGB may have significant effects on appetite, long-term weight loss, and glucose metabolism, but these mechanisms are still being investigated.

The laparoscopic RYGB is performed using five or six trocars. The jejunum is divided 50 cm from the ligament of Treitzanda 150 cm Roux limb is measured. A side-to-side jejunojejunostomy is created and the mesenteric defect closed. A 15–30 ml gastric pouch is created using a linear cutting stapler, thereby completely separating the gastric pouch from the gastric remnant. After dividing the greater omentum, the Roux limb is delivered by most surgeons in an antecolic and antegastric orientation. The retrocolic position can be utilized if necessary to avoid tension on the gastrojejunostomy. The gastrojejunostomy can be created with a hand-sewn technique, a linear stapler, or a circular stapler.

**Advantages:** RYGB is generally a more effective weight loss operation than LAGB and results in 65–80% EWL at 2 years. Several studies have demonstrated 50% EWL 15 years after the operation. RYGB also results in improvement or resolution of obesity-related comorbidities in about 80% of patients, specifically, diabetes, hypertension, dyslipidemia, sleep apnea, asthma, metabolic syndrome, polycystic ovarian syndrome, gout, degenerative joint pain, pseudotumor cerebri, and stress urinary incontinence. Laparoscopic RYGB offers advantages over the open approach with fewer wound complications (incisional hernia, wound infection), fewer pulmonary complications, less postoperative pain, shorter hospital stay, and a faster return to normal activities.

**Complications:** Multiple large series of RYGB have reported perioperative mortality rates from zero to 2%, with the incidence of anastomotic leaks of ~2–5%, bleeding (0–4%), gastrojejunal stenosis (5–15%), marginal ulcers (1–5%), and bowel obstruction (1–10%). Complications requiring reoperation occur in 10–15% of patients after RYGB. Nutritional deficiencies, such as iron-deficiency anemia, vitamin B12 and D deficiencies, and calcium deficiency, can occur in one-third to one-half of patients after RYGB. Routine supplementation after surgery can prevent the majority of these deficiencies but patients require lifelong surveillance of their micronutrient status after gastric bypass.

## Summary

Obesity is a complex disease with genetic, psychosocial, behavioral, and metabolic causes. Current medical therapy does not provide a satisfactory long-term solution for patients with severe obesity. Bariatric surgery is being performed in increasing numbers worldwide as the obesity epidemic grows. A variety of bariatric procedures are performed today and the mechanisms of action, risks, and benefits differ with each. The choice of procedure for a given patient is determined by their own preference, their willingness to accept slightly higher risks for more weight loss (or less weight loss after a lower risk procedure), and the surgeon's experience with specific operations.

Minimally invasive technologies are currently used for most bariatric procedures. Natural orifice transluminal and endoluminal bariatric procedures are being investigated currently. While most of these are in pre-clinical stages of development, the future of bariatric surgery may include endoluminal or transluminal procedures as either primary or adjunctive therapy.

# Selected Readings

Brethauer SA, Chand B, Schauer PR (2006) Risks and benefits of bariatric surgery: Current evidence. Cleve Clin J Med 73:993–1007

Buchwald H, Avidor Y, Braunwald E et al. (2004) Bariatric surgery: a systematic review and meta-analysis. JAMA 292:1724–1737

Chapman AE, Kiroff G, Game P et al. (2004) Laparoscopic adjustable gastric banding in the treatment of obesity: a systematic literature review. Surgery 135:326–351

Christou NV, Sampalis JS, Liberman M et al. (2004) Surgery decreases long-term mortality, morbidity, and health care use in morbidly obese patients. Ann Surg 240:416–423; discussion 423–424

NIH conference (1991) Gastrointestinal surgery for severe obesity. Consensus Development Conference Panel. Ann Intern Med 115:956–961

Ogden CL, Carroll MD, Curtin LR et al. (2006) Prevalence of overweight and obesity in the United States, 1999–2004. JAMA 295:1549–1555

Schauer PR, Burguera B, Ikramuddin S et al. (2003) Effect of laparoscopic Roux-en-Y gastric bypass on type 2 diabetes mellitus. Ann Surg 238:467–484; discussion 84–85

Sjostrom L, Lindroos AK, Peltonen M et al. (2004) Lifestyle, diabetes, and cardiovascular risk factors 10 years after bariatric surgery. N Engl J Med 351:2683–2693

# 17
# Gastric Adenocarcinoma

**Yoshiro Saikawa and Masaki Kitajima**

## Pearls and Pitfalls

- Gastric cancer is one of the most common cancers worldwide.
- Protective factors against gastric carcinoma include dietary intake of fresh fruits and vegetables, vitamin C, and reduction of salt, pickling, and nitrates for food preservation.
- Factors that predispose to gastric cancer include Helicobacter pylori infection, natural carcinogens (e.g., nitrates), carcinogens from meat grilling or barbecuing, and dietary pro-carcinogens.
- Host-related factors associated with an increased risk of gastric adenocarcinoma include low serum ferritin levels and pernicious anemia, distal gastrectomy for benign ulcer, Barrett's esophagus, adenomatous polyps, and heritable and familial risks such as hereditary nonpolyposis colorectal cancer (HNPCC).
- Symptoms, if present, are non-specific for early gastric cancers, while more diagnostic symptoms occur in the advanced cancers.
- Imaging techniques, such as CT, US, EUS, and endoscopy, are helpful in determining appropriate treatment.
- Preoperative laparoscopy is beneficial for detection of peritoneal metastases, liver metastases, or locally advanced, unresectable diseases and may provide avoidance of a non-therapeutic laparotomy.

K.I. Bland et al. (eds.), *Surgery of the Esophagus and Stomach*, DOI: 10.1007/978-1-84996-438-8_17,
© Springer-Verlag London Limited 2011

- Nutritional support through placement of a feeding jejunostomy may be beneficial.
- Staging systems for gastric cancer include: the American Joint Committee on Cancer/Union Internationale Contre le Cancer (AJCC/UICC), the Japanese Classification of Gastric Cancer, the World Health Organization Classification System, and the Lauren Classification System.
- Endoscopic mucosal or submucosal resection may be appropriate for selected patients with early gastric adenocarcinoma.
- Gastrectomy with lymph node dissection is the most widely used curative therapy.
- Surgical options must consider the extent of gastric resection, extent of lymph node dissection, and methods of reconstruction.
- Adjuvant chemotherapy and chemo-radiotherapy with several new drugs, such as CPT-11 and the taxanes, allow palliative control of gastric adenocarcinoma and may prove useful in the neoadjuvant setting.

## Epidemiology and Carcinogenesis

At the beginning of 2000, gastric adenocarcinoma was the second most common cancer worldwide. Although the incidence varies dramatically from country to country, there is a general trend of declining incidence throughout the world, with decreases in gastric adenocarcinoma rates documented in many of the Western nations during the last century. The United States now has one of the lowest rates of gastric cancer in the world. Moreover, a remarkable shift in anatomic location has occurred from noncardia to cardial lesions. The incidences of proximal cardia and gastroesophageal (GE) junction adenocarcinomas have increased in the United States and Europe, suggesting a common pathogenesis distinct from the development of distal gastric carcinomas.

In contrast, the incidence of gastric adenocarcinoma in other countries is alarmingly high. In China, South America,

Eastern Europe, Korea, and Japan, gastric carcinoma is the most common non-skin malignancy. Although most experts generally agree that diet and nutrition play a role in gastric carcinogenesis, the mechanisms that account for the observed patterns of geographic and temporal incidence have not yet been well established. Multiple studies designed to delineate the causes of gastric adenocarcinoma have identified a number of factors that appear to be involved (Table 17.1). Factors that appear to provide a protective role include adequate nutrition, particularly intake of fruit and vegetables, vitamin C intake, and modern techniques of food processing and storage, thereby reducing spoilage and the need for salt-curing, pickling, and nitrates for preservation. In contrast, infection with Helicobacter pylori infection maybe the most important factor worldwide that predisposes patients to gastric cancer.

TABLE 17.1.  Risk factors for gastric cancer.

| Definite-surveillance suggested | Possible |
| --- | --- |
| Familial adenomatous polyposis | Excess alcohol ingestion |
| Gastric adenomas | Gastric hamartomas |
| Gastric biopsy revealing high-grade dysplasia | High intake of salted, pickled, or smoked foods |
| **Definite** | Low intake of fruits and vegetables |
| Chronic atrophic gastritis | Ménétrier's disease |
| Gastric metaplasia on biopsy | Peutz-Jeghers syndrome |
| Helicobacter pylori infection | Tobacco smoking |
| Hereditary nonpolyposis colorectal cancer (Lynch II syndrome) | **Questionable** |
| **Probable** | Benign gastric ulcers |
| History of subtotal gastrectomy (>20 years) | Fundic gland polyps |
| Pernicious anemia | Hyperplastic polyps |
| Tobacco smoking (adenocarcinoma of cardia) | |

Other factors include natural carcinogens or precursors such as nitrates in food, the production of carcinogens during the grilling or barbecuing of meats, and the synthesis of carcinogens from dietary precursors in the stomach.

There are two general types of gastric adenocarcinoma: the intestinal type and the diffuse type. The intestinal type is more common and more often distal in the stomach, while the diffuse type carries a worse prognosis, tends to occur in younger patients, and can arise anywhere in the stomach, but especially in the cardia. Mucosal changes resulting from various kinds of environmental insults can lead eventually to atrophic gastritis, which, when present chronically, can induce intestinal metaplasia that appears to be a precursor state to the intestinal-type gastric adenocarcinoma. Within this setting, various host-related, environmental, and infectious factors have been implicated in the etiology of gastric adenocarcinoma. Host-related factors that may lead to an increased risk of gastric cancer include low serum ferritin levels and pernicious anemia. Although peptic ulcer disease does not appear to be related to increased risk, patients who undergo distal gastrectomy for benign ulcer disease are reported to have a five-fold increased risk of gastric cancer in long-term follow-up. Barrett's esophagus is now accepted as a cause of gastric adenocarcinoma in the distal esophagus and gastric cardia, and adenomatous polyps have been associated with gastric adenocarcinoma. With regard to the risk of inheritable gastric adenocarcinoma, patients with hereditary nonpolyposis colorectal cancer (HNPCC) have an increased risk of gastric adenocarcinoma, while patients with familial adenomatous polyposis do not have a similar risk. In terms of environmental causes, food refrigeration has probably decreased the dietary exposure to various carcinogens, such as nitrates and nitrites, by reducing the bacterial and fungal contamination of food. Refrigeration has also led to a decrease in consumption of smoked, cured, and salted foods, thereby reducing the incidence of intestinal-type gastric adenocarcinoma. A higher intake of fruits and vegetables is known to be protective against gastric carcinogenesis, while a modest increase in risk has been reported for increased meat consumption, with a positive correlation with longer cooking times. Other environmental factors, such as smoking or industrial dust exposure, may also be associated with gastric adenocarcinoma. Chronic infections of the stomach, such as by *Helicobacter pylori* (HP) or Epstein-Barr virus, have been implicated repeatedly in epidemiologic studies, and a relationship between chronic infection and gastric carcinogenesis has been suggested by various studies.

# Clinical Diagnosis and Pathologic Staging

## *Clinical Presentation*

The symptoms of gastric cancer are often non-specific, usually without obvious symptoms during early stages, and often with only few or minimal symptoms that lead to diagnosis even at advanced stages. Due to the relatively large size of the stomach and abdominal cavity, mechanical symptoms such as obstruction or hemorrhage caused by a tumor mass are recognized only rarely until the tumor becomes large unless it is in the distal antrum. Non-specific symptoms, such as vague gastrointestinal distress, episodic nausea, vomiting, and anorexia, are common in patients without cancer and are often not taken seriously by the patient or physician, unless the symptoms are severe or progressive. Common symptoms at diagnosis are abdominal pain and weight loss. Although anemia is a frequent finding in gastric cancer patients, substantive upper gastrointestinal bleeding is uncommon. At advanced stages, proximally localized esophageal dysphasia is observed frequently, while nausea and/or vomiting maybe due to circumferential involvement of either the stomach or the cardia that leads to mechanical obstruction.

Findings on physical examination, such as a palpable mass, jaundice (lymph node involvement in hepatoduodenal ligaments) or a Blumer's shelf (pelvic peritoneal metastasis), Krukenberg tumors (in ovaries), or periumbilical masses (peritoneal metastases) tend to occur in highly advanced, unresectable disease. Palpable lymphadenopathy of the left supraclavicular fossa (Virchow's node) can sometimes be observed without other complaints. Less common dermatologic findings include acanthosis nigricans and multiple seborrheic keratoses.

## Clinical Staging with Imaging

To confirm the clinical staging of a gastric adenocarcinoma, patients should be evaluated in a stepwise fashion with physical examination, laboratory studies, computerized tomography (CT), endoscopic ultrasonography (EUS), and often, staging laparoscopy.

Physical examination should be directed toward evaluation of nutritional and performance states and detecting evidence of distant spread. Palpations for adenopathy in the supraclavicular fossa (Virchow node), the periumbilical area (Sister Mary Joseph node), and the left axilla (Irish node) are indicative of unresectable disease. The abdomen should be examined for the presence of palpable masses or ascites. A digital rectal exam may be performed to assess for masses or a Blumer's shelf in the pelvis. Laboratory studies should include complete blood count, electrolytes, blood urea nitrogen, and serum creatinine, as well as liver function tests. Tumor markers, such as carcinoembryonic antigen and CA 19-9, should be obtained to predict cancer state and malignant potential.

CT of the abdomen, pelvis, and chest (for proximal lesions) should be performed to evaluate the primary gastric neoplasm and to look for liver metastases, ascites, peritoneal nodules, and nodal metastases to allow assessment of clinical stage. EUS can be useful to assess both tumor T-stage and regional nodes. Endoscopy, CT, and EUS should be performed to confirm clinical staging. Accurate staging is imperative to guide the appropriate therapeutic strategy for gastric adenocarcinoma, ranging from endoscopic or laparoscopic intervention for early cancer to neoadjuvant or palliative chemotherapy for highly advanced malignancy.

Staging laparoscopy may be essential for complete staging and evaluation of peritoneal metastases, especially for patients with potentially resectable gastric cancer based on preoperative imaging and endoscopy. A feeding tube jejunostomy can also be placed during the staging laparoscopy; however, in the presence of ascites, the benefits of a jejunostomy tube should be considered carefully against the risks of abdominal and jejunostomy site complications.

## Clinico-Pathologic Staging Systems

*The AJCC/UICC System in Pathologic Staging* (Tables 17.2 and 17.3): The American Joint Committee on Cancer/Union Internationale Contrele Cancer (AJCC/UICC) system is the most widely used pathologic staging system for gastric cancer and evaluates the primary tumor (T), regional lymph nodes (N), and distant metastatic disease (M). T stage is divided into

TABLE 17.2. TNM definition.

Primary tumor (T)

- TX: Primary tumor cannot be assessed

- T0: No evidence of primary tumor

- Tis: Carcinoma in situ: intraepithelial tumor without invasion of the lamina propria

- T1: Tumor invades lamina propria or submucosa

- T2: Tumor invades the muscularis propria or the subserosa[a]

- T2a: Tumor invades muscularis propria

- T2b: Tumor invades subserosa

- T3: Tumor penetrates the serosa (visceral peritoneum) without invading adjacent structures[b,c]

- T4: Tumor invades adjacent structures[b,c]

- Regional lymph nodes (N)

(*continued*)

TABLE 17.2. (continued).

- Regional lymph nodes include perigastric nodes found along lesser and greater curvatures and nodes located along left gastric, common hepatic, splenic, and celiac arteries. For pN, a regional lymphadenectomy specimen will ordinarily contain at least 15 lymph nodes. Involvement of other intra-abdominal lymph nodes, such as hepatoduodenal, retropancreatic, mesenteric, and para-aortic, is classified as distant metastasis.

- NX: Regional lymph node(s) cannot be assessed

- N0: No regional lymph node metastasis[d]

- N1: Metastasis in 1–6 regional lymph nodes

- N2: Metastasis in 7–15 regional lymph nodes

- N3: Metastasis in more than 15 regional lymph nodes

- Distant metastasis (M)

MX: Distant metastasis cannot be assessed

M0: No distant metastasis

M1: Distant metastasis

[a]Note: A tumor may penetrate muscularis propria with extension into gastrocolic or gastrohepatic ligaments, or into greater or lesser omentum, without extension through visceral peritoneum covering these structures. In this case, the tumor is classified T2. If there is extension through visceral peritoneum covering gastric ligaments or omentum, the tumor should be classified T3.

[b]Note: Adjacent structures of the stomach include spleen, transverse colon, liver, diaphragm, pancreas, abdominal wall, adrenal gland, kidney, small intestine, and retroperitoneum.

[c]Note: Intramural extension to the duodenum or esophagus is classified by the depth of greatest invasion in any of these sites, including stomach.

[d]Note: A designation of pN0 should be used if all examined lymph nodes are negative, regardless of total number removed and examined.

TABLE 17.3.  AJCC stage groupings.

Stage 0

- Tis, N0, M0

Stage IA

- T1, N0, M0

Stage IB

- T1, N1, M0
- T2a, N0, M0
- T2b, N0, M0

Stage II

- T1, N2, M0
- T2a, N1, M0
- T2b, N1, M0
- T3, N0, M0

Stage IIIA

- T2a, N2, M0
- T2b, N2, M0
- T3, N1, M0
- T4, N0, M0

Stage IIIB

- T3, N2, M0

Stage IV

- T4, N1, M0
- T4, N2, M0
- T4, N3, M0
- T1, N3, M0
- T2, N3, M0
- T3, N3, M0
- Any T, any N, M1

four levels based on the depth of penetration into the stomach wall. T1 tumors are the most superficial, with involvement only as deep as the submucosa. T2 tumors invade into the muscularis propria, and T3 tumors are into the serosa. T2 tumors are divided into T2a (invasion of the muscularis propria) and T2b (invasion of the subserosa). T4 tumors invade adjacent organs directly. N stage is divided into four levels based on the number of positive local lymph nodes: N0 = 0; N1 = 1–6; N2 = 7–15; N3 = >15, no longer on the site of nodal metastases. Patients with N3 nodal disease are classified as stage IV.

The classification of gastric carcinoma reported by the Japanese Research Society of Gastric Cancer defines nodal stage by anatomic location and proximity to the primary tumor, based on the division of six perigastric stations (right and left cardia, lesser and greater curvatures, and supra and infra pyloric), and five additional stations along the celiac vessels (celiac, hepatic, left gastric, splenic, hilum of the spleen). While the AJCC/UICC N staging was based on the Japanese system, proximity to the tumor may not necessarily reflect prognostic value in terms of nodal staging.

*Lauren Classification System*: The Lauren system is another major classification system for gastric adenocarcinoma that divides the disease into intestinal and diffuse types; however, cancers with a mixed histology containing components of both intestinal and diffuse disease have been described. Intestinal-type gastric cancer is also called the "epidemic" type, because it retains glandular structures and cellular polarity. Grossly, the intestinal type usually has a sharp margin, arises from the gastric mucosa, and is associated with chronic gastritis, gastric atrophy, and intestinal metaplasia. Helicobacter pylori and other environmental factors are thought to play major roles in its pathogenesis. The diffuse-type histology is associated with an invasive growth pattern with scattered clusters of uniformly-sized malignant cells that frequently infiltrate the submucosa. This diffuse type has little glandular formation, and mucin production is common. The infiltrative growth pattern observed in diffuse-type gastric cancers often leads to cancers without a mass and present as advanced linitis plastica. Endoscopically, such cancers may be difficult to identify without ulceration or mass formation. For example, linitis plastica is observed as a non-distensible, leather bottle-like appearance on the stomach.

*World Health Organization Classification System*: The World Health Organization (WHO) scheme divides Lauren intestinal-type gastric adenocarcinomas into papillary or tubular groups, and the Lauren diffuse-type into mucinous or signet ring cell groups. While this system is not frequently utilized worldwide, it offers more information than smaller classification schemes for gastric adenocarcinoma.

# Treatment

## Endoscopic Mucosal Resection and Endoscopic Submucosal Dissection

Techniques of endoscopic mucosal resection (EMR) for mucosal (M) cancer of the stomach are based on similar endoscopic techniques for resection of colonic polyps, while endoscopic techniques of submucosal dissection (ESD) have been developed recently for the treatment of T1 gastric adenocarcinoma and submucosal cancer (SM). Cure by endoscopic treatment of T1 tumors (M or SM tumors) maybe achieved in patients without evidence of residual cancer or nodal disease. While the presence of nodal metastases is approximately 10% for T1 gastric adenocarcinomas, M cancers have a 1–3% incidence of positive nodes and SM cancers have an incidence of around 15%. Risk of nodal positivity is increased in patients with Borrmann tumor classification types 3–5, poorly differentiated or signet ring cell neoplasms, evidence of lymphatic invasion, or large tumor size (>2.0 cm).

In Japan, more than half of patients with gastric adenocarcinoma have early (T1) gastric cancer. This finding has been attributed to the use of sophisticated social education and mass screening programs. Endoscopic treatment has been performed successfully for T1 cancers, especially M gastric adenocarcinomas, while operative intervention is recommended for SM invasion, venous or lymphatic invasion, or positive margins after endoscopic resection. Worldwide, the use of minimally invasive procedures is dependent on economically appropriate costs and the health and welfare policies of each country.

# Operative Indications and Curative Operations

Patient comorbidities should be reviewed when considering operative resection. Intervention is indicated when resection enables a beneficial outcome for the patient, aiming at either cure or palliation to improve quality of life (QOL). While recent developments in anticancer drugs and interventional endoscopic techniques have allowed control of tumor bleeding or mechanical obstruction in many patients with advanced gastric adenocarcinoma, palliative bypass or resection maybe an option in selected patients.

When intervention is intended for cure, the extent of gastric resection, lymphadenectomy, role of splenectomy, and method of reconstruction should be determined according to location and histologic type of the neoplasm, as well as the disease stage. Gastrectomy remains the only treatment of invasive gastric cancer offering long-term survival.

Several prospective and randomized studies have failed to demonstrate a survival advantage of total gastrectomy compared with distal subtotal gastrectomy. Additionally, QOL after subtotal gastrectomy is superior to that after total gastrectomy. These findings have led to the preference for subtotal gastrectomy when an adequate margin can be obtained distant from the primary neoplasm.

The issue of lymph node dissection remains controversial in the surgical management of gastric adenocarcinoma. The extent of lymph node dissection is defined by the D (dissection) designation; D1 dissection includes only perigastric lymph nodes, while a D2 dissection also includes nodes along the named gastric arteries, including the hepatic, left gastric, celiac, and splenic arteries, and those in the splenic hilum. Dissections which include nodes along the porta hepatis, retropancreatic, and periaortic areas are classified as D3.

Although retrospective studies from Japan suggest that extended lymphadenectomy can improve survival in patients with stage II or III disease with perioperative mortality rates of 1%, a Dutch prospective, randomized multi-center trial showed higher patient operative morbidity and mortality after D2 compared with D1 resections (43% and 10% vs.25% and 4%,respectively, p < 0.01 each). Subset analysis (post hoc) of this latter study showed that survival of patients with stage II or IIIA disease was better after a D2 dissection, but the study was not powered to address this question adequately. The overall survival benefit of extended lymph node dissection may be around 5–8%, but obligates considerable operative morbidity and mortality rates, when splenectomy or distal pancreatectomy (to aid the lymphadenectomy) is performed. D3 lymph node dissections may be considered by experienced surgeons with excellent technique and low operative morbidity and mortality rates. Data from the American College of Surgeons indicate that the risk of mortality with a D3 resection is in the range of 8–9% across the United States, and thus D3 resections cannot be recommended routinely.

When necessary to achieve an R0 resection, resections of involved adjacent organs (colon, diaphragm, liver, pancreas) should be considered in centers with low operative mortality rates. The risk of mortality is increased to 15% when distal pancreatectomy and splenectomy are performed as concomitant procedures during gastrectomy in low volume hospitals.

Options for reconstruction after total gastrectomy include the standard Roux-en-Y esophago-jejunostomy, construction of a jejunal pouch, or jejunal interposition (with or without a pouch). While each of these approaches has its advocates, there are no large, controlled trials demonstrating superiority of one approach over the other. The most common reconstruction after total gastrectomy remains a simple esophago-jejunostomy to a Roux-en-Y limb, and in the absence of any conclusive data, it can be argued that the simpler procedure is probably the best. For subtotal gastrectomy, reconstruction options include a Billroth I-like gastroduodenostomy, a loop reconstruction (Billroth II), a jejunal inter-position, and a Roux-en-Y reconstruction. The choice depends on gastroduodenal mobility as well as the size/volume of the gastric remnant; small gastric remnants are best drained by a Roux-en-Y limb to prevent bile reflux esophagitis after a B-II-type drainage. The anastomosis should be large enough to provide optimal emptying of the gastric remnant. The gastro-jejunostomy can be constructed utilizing a circular or linear stapler or by a hand-sewn technique. Debate continues with regard to anastomotic stricture and leak rates among the various techniques (stapler vs. hand-sewn).

## Chemotherapy and Chemoradiotherapy for Gastric Cancer

Single agent treatments of 5-fluorouracil (5-FU), doxorubicin (DXR), mitomycin C (MMC), or cisplatin (CDDP) provide partial response rates of 10–30%. Response rates with 5-FU of up to 20% have been reported and with only mild toxicity. An oral "pro-drug" form of 5-FU composed of uracil and tegafur (UFT) has demonstrated a response rate of 28%, with a median survival of 6 months. When administered orally, UFT is tolerated better than 5-FU. Another oral 5-FU pro-drug currently under clinical trial is S-1, a combination of tegafur and 5-chloro-2, 4-dihydropyrimidine (a dihydropyrimidine dehydrogenase inhibitor) and oteracil (anti-diarrhea). This drug has been evaluated in two Japanese Phase II trials for gastric cancer and showed response rates of 44–49% with a median survival of 7–8 months. While the results for S-1 are promising, further study in larger confirmatory trials is required.

Cisplatin (CDDP), a metal (platinum) with broad-spectrum, anti-tumor activity, offers response rates of 19–33%. Carboplatin, an analog of CDDP with less renal toxicity, has little activity as a single agent against gastric cancer, with only a 5% response rate, but a novel CDDP analog, oxaliplatin, is also now being studied. The topoisomerase I inhibitor irinotecan had a 23% response rate in a phase II trial. Microtubule agents known as taxanes (paclitaxel and docetaxel) have exhibited overall response rates of 17% for paclitaxel and 17–24% for docetaxel.

To improve overall survival and response rates, a number of combination chemotherapy programs have been investigated based on agents with known activity. Numerous patients have been treated with FAM (5-FU plus doxorubicin and mitomycin) since 1980, offering a 30% overall response rate and a 2% complete response rate. To increase the activity of 5-FU-based regimens, doxorubicin and methotrexate, along with 5-FU (FAMTX), have increased the response rate to 58%, with a complete remission rate of 12%; however, this regimen confers a relatively high mortality rate (3%). Nonetheless, the EORTC showed superiority of FAMTX to FAM in terms of response rate (45% vs.9%, p < 0.0001), and median survival (10.5 months vs. 7 months).

Etoposide, doxorubicin, and cisplatin (EAP) were used in a Phase II trial for patients with advanced gastric cancer and gave a response rate of 64% (95% CI, 52% to 76%) and a complete remission rate of 21%; however, three subsequent Phase II trials of EAP showed excessive treatment-related mortality(6% to 14%) despite good efficacy (response rates: 43–72%). Subsequently, EAP and FAMTX were compared in a randomized Phase II trial that also observed excessive toxicities and treatment-related deaths (13%) for the EAP group.

Combined epirubicin, cisplatin, and 5-FU (ECF) have also been compared with FAMTX in a phase III trial. ECF had a greater response rate of 46% (95% CI, 37–55%), compared with 21% (95% CI, 13–28%) for the FAMTX group. In addition, ECF resulted in a superior median survival (9 vs. 6 for FAMTX, p = 0.0005). The combination of etoposide, leucovorin, and 5-FU (ELF) was assessed by the EORTC as part of a three-arm, randomized trial of FAMTX, ELF, and 5-FU plus CDDP, and showed response rates of 12%, 9%, and 20%, respectively, but with similar 7-month median survival times for all three groups.

To investigate combination chemotherapies based on the novel drugs irinotecan and cisplatin, several Phase I/II studies have been conducted using different regimens. The response rates of these trials were 42–58%, suggesting that such regimens maybe effective in palliating gastric adenocarcinoma. Similarly, when the recently developed taxane drugs paclitaxel and docetaxel were added to a 5-FU and cisplatin regimen, a 51% objective response was achieved (95% CI, 37–66%).

Docetaxel-based chemotherapy regimens have also been studied extensively for gastric adenocarcinoma. Phase II trials using combined docetaxel and cisplatin had response rates of 33–56%, with median survival durations of 9–10 months. In addition, the combination of docetaxel, CDDP, and 5-FU (DCF) showed high response rates of 52–56% and is considered currently one of the best regimens. Japanese investigators recently tested the combination of S-1 and CDDP in a Phase I/II trial and demonstrated a response rate of 76%.

Radiation therapy is known to be effective against gastrointestinal cancers including gastric adenocarcinoma, but remains somewhat controversial in neoadjuvant and adjuvant settings. Because the sensitivity spectrum of chemotherapy may be different from that of radiotherapy, adjuvant radiotherapy may be effective against chemo-resistant cells that survive chemotherapy, as suggested by one American trial.

# Selected Readings

Bonenkamp JJ, Hermans J, Sasako M, Velde van de CJ (1999) Extended lymph node dissection for gastric cancer. Dutch Gastric Cancer Group. NEJM 340:908–914

Bruckner HW, Morris JC, Mansfield P (2003) In: Kufe DW, Pollock RE, Weichselbaum RR et al. (eds) Cancer medicine, 6th edn. BC Decker, Ontario

Hans-Olov A, Hunter D, Trichopoulos D et al. (2002) A textbook of cancer epidemiology, 1st edn. Oxford University Press, New York

Houghton J, Stoicov C, Nomura S et al. (2004) Gastric cancer originating from bone marrow-derived cells. Science 306:1568–1571

Japanese Research Society for Gastric Cancer (1995) Japanese classification of gastric carcinoma, First English edition. Kanehara, Tokyo

Mullaney PJ, Wadley MS, Hyde C et al. (2002) Appraisal of compliance with the UICC/AJCC staging system in the staging of gastric cancer. Union International Contra la Cancrum/American Joint Committee on Cancer. Br J Surg 89:1405–1408

Rustgi AK (2000) Neoplasms of the stomach. In: Cecil RL, Goldman L, Bennett JC (eds) Cecil textbook of medicine, 21st edn. W. B. Saunders, Philadelphia, pp. 738–741

# 18
# Gastrointestinal Stromal Tumors

**Francesco P. Prete and Ronald P. DeMatteo**

## Pearls and Pitfalls

- Gastrointestinal stromal tumor (GIST) is the most common mesenchymal neoplasm of the GI tract, while other intestinal sarcomas (lipoma, leiomyoma, and leiomyosarcoma) are infrequent.
- GIST is diagnosed by a combination of cellular morphology on hematoxylin-eosin staining and KIT immunohistochemistry. Rarely, GIST does not overexpress KIT and molecular evaluation may be necessary to render the diagnosis.
- Complete surgical resection is the standard treatment for primary, localized GIST and regional lymph nodes are involved rarely.
- The clinical behavior of GIST is variable, but nearly all lesions have the potential to behave in a malignant fashion (i.e., metastasize). The risk of GIST recurrence is increased with a mitotic rate > 5/50 high power fields, tumor size > 5 cm, and intestinal (vs. stomach) origin.
- The majority of GISTs have a mutation in the *KIT* proto-oncogene, or occasionally in *PDGFRα*, and effective tyrosine kinase inhibitors have been developed against both associated proteins.
- In metastatic GIST, imatinib mesylate (Gleevec) achieves stable disease or a partial response in over 75% of patients and is continued unless there is intolerance or resistance

K.I. Bland et al. (eds.), *Surgery of the Esophagus and Stomach*, DOI: 10.1007/978-1-84996-438-8_18,
© Springer-Verlag London Limited 2011

(progression). The median time of acquired resistance to imatinib is less than 2 years. Sunitinib (Sutent) is a second line agent.

- There may be benefit of resecting metastatic GIST that is stable on tyrosine kinase inhibitor (TKI) therapy.
- The value of imatinib as an adjuvant treatment is under investigation.

# Presentation

Gastrointestinal stromal tumor (GIST) accounts for approximately 80% of all GI mesenchymal tumors. Originally considered to derive from smooth muscle, and variably classified as GI leio-myoma or leiomyosarcoma on the basis of light microscopy appearance, GIST was recognized widely as a distinct disease in the last decade, with the advent of immunohistochemical staining and ultrastructural evaluation. Currently, GIST is defined as a KIT-expressing or KIT-signaling driven primary spindle cell or epithelioid mesenchymal neoplasm of the GI tract, commonly harboring an activating mutation in either the KIT (italics denotes the gene as opposed to the protein) or platelet-derived growth factor receptor alpha (PDGFRα) gene, both of which encode for receptor tyrosine kinases.

## Pathogenesis

KIT is a proto-oncogene that encodes for a transmembrane receptor glycoprotein with tyrosine kinase function. The KIT protein is expressed commonly by the intestinal interstitial pacemaker cells of Cajal (from which GISTs are believed to derive), hematopoietic cells, mast cells, and germ cells. KIT functions in differentiation, cell growth, and survival. In up to 90% of GISTs, a single gain-of function mutation is present in the KIT gene, leading to constitutive, ligand-independent activation of the receptor tyrosine kinase function. The most frequent sites of *KIT* mutation are in exon 11 of the gene (70%), which codes for the juxtamembrane domain of the KIT protein, or in exon 9 (10%). Exons 13 and 17 are rarely involved. KIT protein is expressed by the overwhelming majority (95%) of GISTs, and the antigenic determinant of the receptor (CD117 antigen) can be detected with simple immunohistochemical staining. A small subset of GISTs (5%) with otherwise typical clinicopathologic and cytogenetic features do not express detectable KIT protein and are CD117 negative. In a fraction of GISTs (approximately 3%), mutation occurs in *PDGFRα* but not *KIT*. *PDGFRα* mutation usually involves exon 12 (intracellular juxtamembrane region) or exon 18 (activation loop). These sites correspond to the *KIT* exons containing oncogenic mutations in many GISTs, and the downstream activation of intracellular intermediates and the cytogenetic changes occurring with tumor progression are similar to those from GISTs with *KIT* mutation. Overall, about 10% of all GISTs do not have a detectable mutation in either *KIT* or *PDGFRα* and are designated as wild-type with an unknown molecular pathogenesis. The presence of the constitutively activated mutant *KIT* isoforms (and some of the mutant *PDGFRα* isoforms) is clinically important, because the tumors are sensitive to the selective tyrosine kinase inhibiting agent imatinib mesylate, validating the molecularly targeted approach to cancer therapy.

## Incidence and Anatomical Distribution

GIST is the most common mesenchymal neoplasm of the GI tract, but accounts for less than 1% of GI malignant neoplasms. The incidence is approximately 15 cases per million, with a prevalence of 129 cases per million. GIST represents about 20% of small-bowel malignant neoplasms (excluding lymphoma), 1–2% of gastric malignancies, and less than 1% of malignancies involving the esophagus, colon, and rectum. No racial predilection exists. Men are affected slightly more often than women. The majority of patients are between 40 and 80 years of age at the time of diagnosis (median 60 years), but the disease spans over a broad spectrum of age. GIST occurs rarely in adolescents or children. Approximately 60% of GIST occurs in the stomach, usually in the fundus. About 30% of tumors occur in the small intestine, and are most commonly found in the jejunum, followed by the ileum and the duodenum. Another 1–5% arise in the esophagus, and 5% are located in the colon and rectum. On rare occasions, GIST develops outside the gastrointestinal tract in the mesentery, omentum, or retro-peritoneum. GISTs are multicentric in fewer than 5% of cases. Rarely GISTs (mainly gastric, involving the body and the antrum) may occur in association with functioning extra-adrenal paraganglioma and pulmonary chondroma in the context of "Carney's triad", a rare syndrome of unknown etiology reported in young women. GISTs arising in this setting, even if metastatic, characteristically have a slower and more indolent clinical course than sporadic cases. These patients are wild-type for KIT and *PDGFRα*. GISTs related to the Neurofibromatosis type-1 syndrome seem to rely on the activation of alternative kinase pathways, and again the patients are wild-type for KIT and *PDGFRα*. KIT or *PDGFRα* germline mutations have been detected in at least a dozen kindreds with familial GIST in the world.

## Clinical Features

There is a broad range of possible patient presentations in GIST. In the majority (about 70%) of cases, patients will seek medical attention because of nonspecific symptoms: nausea, early satiety, vomiting, abdominal discomfort, or vague abdominal pain. These symptoms reflect the typical growth pattern of GIST which, similar to other sarcomas, tends to displace but not invade adjacent structures. Consequently, a GIST is often clinically silent until it becomes large. Occasionally, an increase in abdominal girth or a palpable mass may be present. Overall, the mean duration of symptoms is 4–6 months. Small tumors (usually within 2–3 cm) are more likely to be incidentally detected in asymptomatic patients on radiologic imaging, abdominal exploration, or endoscopy. GIST may result in ulceration of the gut mucosa. After initial growth as a submucosal mass, GIST may then erode into the lumen of the intestinal tract and produce gastrointestinal bleeding. Blood loss is usually subclinical and may produce fatigue and microcytic anemia. However, up to 25% of patients present with acute GI hemorrhage. Large tumors that outgrow their blood supply may become necrotic and rupture into the peritoneal cavity, resulting in life-threatening hemorrhage. Other symptoms are particular to the site of tumor origin, so an esophageal GIST may cause dysphagia, or a rare periampullary GIST may result in biliary obstruction. Intestinal obstruction is uncommon; the tumor can act rarely as a lead point for intussusception. In the rectum, GISTs usually present as small, hard nodules less than 1 cm in diameter found incidentally during clinical examination. Large tumors can ulcerate and may mimic a rectal adenocarcinoma. The clinical behavior of any particular GIST is difficult to predict. With prolonged follow-up, it appears that almost any GIST presenting with clinical symptoms or signs leading to treatment has the potential to behave in a malignant fashion. On presentation, about 25% of GISTs have already metastasized. Metastases most commonly involve the liver, omentum, and the peritoneal cavity. Dissemination to the lungs and to extra-abdominal organs usually occurs late in the course of disease.

# Diagnosis

## *Initial Assessment*

The clinical diagnosis of GIST requires a high level of suspicion, as the patient's history and physical examination are usually nonspecific. Abdominal imaging (ultrasound, CT scan, or MRI) is usually performed because of a mass, abdominal pain, or other symptoms, and it is important to define the characteristics of a gastrointestinal mass, evaluate resectability, and determine distant spread of the disease. The possibility of a GIST should be considered when a circumscribed, vascular, exophytic mass is found in relation to the stomach or the intestine.

## Cross-Sectional Imaging

Contrast-enhanced CT is useful to confirm and characterize an abdominal mass related to the gut. Oral and IV contrast should be administered to properly define the bowel margins. At CT scan, smaller GISTs present typically as hyperdense, well-defined solid masses with homogeneous attenuation, with uniform or rim-like bright enhancement after IV contrast. Occasionally, dense focal calcifications are present. Large tumors (>10 cm) present usually with enhancing borders of variable thickness and may contain irregular central areas of fluid as a result of necrosis or hemorrhage. In the majority of cases, the tumor margin appears smooth or lobular. The vessels surrounding large masses can appear stretched, but encasement is uncommon. CT can detect the presence or absence of metastatic disease in the liver, lungs, bone, and peritoneum. Liver metastases tend to appear hypodense in the portal phase but are hypervascular in the arterial phase.

MR imaging is useful for a low rectal mass or when the patient is intolerant to CT scan contrast. GIST appears isointense on T1-weighted and hyperintense on T2-weighted images, and again takes up contrast.

## Upper Endoscopy

Endoscopy may be useful to characterize a gastric or duodenal lesion further. Small GISTs typically appear as a submucosal mass with smooth margins and a normal overlying mucosa. Sometimes they bulge into the gastric lumen and central ulceration is seen occasionally. Endoscopic ultrasound can be useful to define the local extension of a tumor incidentally discovered during endoscopy. However, sonographic characteristics alone provide insufficient information to assess the clinical behavior of the tumor.

## Biopsy

If a suspected GIST appears resectable, preoperative biopsy is not required, because GISTs are soft and fragile and can easily bleed or rupture resulting in tumor dissemination. Most pathologists cannot reliably render a diagnosis of GIST from a percutaneous biopsy, especially when only a fine-needle aspirate is obtained or a necrotic portion of the tumor is sampled. The chance of bleeding or rupture is minimal in the case of endoscopic biopsy. A biopsy is preferred to confirm the diagnosis if metastatic disease is suspected, if there is a possibility that the diagnosis may be lymphoma, or if preoperative imatinib is considered prior to attempted resection in a patient who has a large locally advanced lesion thought to represent a GIST.

## Pathologic Diagnosis

The diagnosis of GIST relies on the presence of characteristic morphologic findings on hematoxylin-eosin staining and the expression of the KIT receptor on immunohistochemistry, with central review by an expert in sarcoma pathology for equivocal cases. Three main morphologic types of GIST exist: spindle (70%), epithelioid (20%), and mixed spindle and epithelioid (10%). GIST tends to have bland morphologic features, which per se are not predictive of biologic behavior. CD117 immunohistochemistry is positive in up to 95% of cases, CD34 in 70% of cases, smooth muscle actin in 40%, S-100 in 5%, while desmin is mostly negative (2% of cases). KIT staining is generally intense and diffuse in GIST. Immunohistochemical examination is performed usually without antigen retrieval, as this can result in false positive staining for CD117. Molecular analysis for *KIT* or *PDGFRα* mutation is performed in cases of weak or absent CD117 staining, since this may occur in KIT-negative GISTs or other types of tumors. The optimal method for mutational analysis is still to be defined. Mutations in *KIT* exon 9 are typically of small intestine origin, while *PDGFRα* exon 18 mutations are typical of stomach and omental GISTs. The karyotype of GIST is characterized frequently by the deletions in chromosomes 14, 22 and 1p. The clinical behavior is variable. All GISTs are regarded as potentially malignant, with the possible exception of very small (<1 cm) tumors, and it seems appropriate to stratify GISTs according to their risk of progression rather than as benign or malignant. There is general consensus that mitotic rate, tumor size, and tumor site are the most important predictors (Table 18.1). Gastric GIST tendst to have a more favorable outcome than GIST of the small intestine. GIST with exon 9 mutation appears to be more aggressive than those with exon 11 mutation. No significant correlation has been shown between survival and sex, or intensity or distribution of the staining for CD117. The prognostic significance of grading in GISTs is not clear.

# Treatment

## *Primary Localized Disease That is Resectable*

The management of GIST depends upon the confidence in the preoperative diagnosis, tumor location, size, and clinical presentation (Fig. 18.1). Since almost every GIST is

TABLE 18.1. Estimation of malignant potential of GIST (Adapted from Miettinen et al., 2002, copyright 2002. With permission from Elsevier).

|  | Gastric | | Intestinal | |
|---|---|---|---|---|
|  | Size (cm) | Mitoses per 50 HPF | Size (cm) | Mitoses per 50 HPF |
| Likely benign | ≤5 | ≤5 | ≤2 | ≤5 |
| Intermediate | 5–10 | ≤5 | 2–5 | ≤5 |
| Probably malignant | >10 | >5 | >5 | >5 |

*HPF – high power fields.*

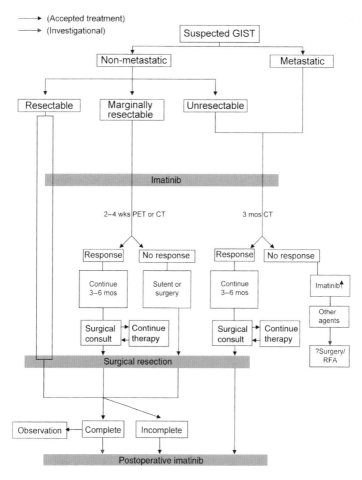

FIGURE 18.1. Summary of present treatment and investigational pathway of gastrointestinal stromal tumor.

considered to have malignant potential, nearly all of them should be resected. The management of small (<1 cm) tumors is unclear. The standard therapy for primary GIST is complete surgical resection. In the pre-imatinib era, the median survival was 66 months in patients who underwent complete gross resection of the primary disease and only 22 months in patients with incomplete or unresectable primary tumors. At laparotomy, the abdomen should be explored thoroughly, withwparticulartattention to the peritoneal surfaces and the liver to exclude metastatic spread. Wedge resection of the stomach or segmental resection of the small intestine should be performed as opposed to wide resections. Although many primary GISTs may appear ominous on CT, they can often be lifted away from surrounding structures, since they tend to displace rather than invade adjacent organs. However, in case of dense adhesions, an en bloc resection should be considered. When a tumor arises in the esophagus, duodenum or rectum, where wedge resection may not be feasible, preference should be given to a wide resection. In extra-gastrointestinal GISTs (mesentery or omentum), en bloc complete resection of all the visible disease should be performed, encompassing any adherent organs. Intraoperative violation of the tumor pseudocapsule increases the risk of peritoneal recurrence and should be avoided. Thus, the tumor should be handled carefully, and meticulous surgical technique is necessary, because GISTs are soft and fragile. In general, every effort should be made to achieve negative resection margins, as positive margins may result in a higher risk of peritoneal relapse. It seems appropriate to consider re-excision after previous surgery with positive margins, but the risks and benefits of re-excision versus watchful waiting must be considered carefully. The management of a positive microscopic margin on the final pathology report depends also on whether the surgeon believes the finding reflects accurately the surgical procedure that was undertaken; for example, if a wedge resection was performed with a surgical stapler, the pathologist may not interpret the margin correctly once the staple line is cut away. Re-excision should also be considered following endoscopic removal of a GIST. The importance of negative surgical margins is uncertain for large GISTs, which may shed tumor cells into the peritoneum from anywhere along their surface. Since nodal metastases are rare, lymph node dissection is indicated only when nodal metastases are suspected. Often what is considered to be a lymph node is actually a satellite peritoneal metastasis. Laparoscopic resection of GIST is possible by experienced surgeons. Generally, laparoscopy should only be used for tumors < 5 cm to minimize intraoperative rupture.

## Primary Localized Disease That is Not Resectable

The first-line treatment for patients with unresectable GIST (because of tumor proximity to important neurovascular structures, or risk of important functional consequences after resection of surrounding organs) is imatinib mesylate. If a GIST responds to imatinib and appears resectable, then surgery may be possible. CT scan is the preferred method to assess treatment response to imatinib. A scan is performed typically after 1 month of therapy to make sure that the patient is not in the 15% of patients who are resistant primarily to imatinib. In that case, sunitinib may be tried. Sufficient tumor shrinkage on either agent can require 6 or more months of therapy.

## Primary Disease with Metastasis

In general, patients with a primary GIST and synchronous metastasis should be treated first with imatinib, even when all disease is technically removable. The exceptions include those with a low volume of metastatic disease or patients with symptoms.

## Metastatic Disease

In patients presenting with metastatic disease, the first-line treatment is imatinib. Up to 80% of patients with metastatic GIST achieve a partial response or stable disease while receiving imatinib. Data from the pre-imatinib era demonstrate that surgical treatment alone of metastatic GIST almost never results in cure. Therefore, if resection becomes feasible, imatinib should be continued after surgery.

## Imatinib Mesylate

Imatinib is a multi-kinase inhibitor, which acts on the tyrosine kinase BCR-ABL (involved in chronic myeloid leukemia) and on the protein kinases KIT and PDGFRα. The mechanism of inhibition is competitive. Competing with ATP for the binding to the catalytic site of the receptor, imatinib blocks the transfer of a phosphate group to the substrate, and therefore blocks the transduction of the signals generated by the activation of KIT or PDGFRα.

Imatinib should be started at the diagnosis of unresectable or metastatic GIST. The general starting dose of imatinib is 400 mg/day, although one study suggests a longer progression-free survival at a dose of 800 mg/day. In general, an increase of dose is not recommended in cases of stable disease. The dose can be increased if progression occurs after an initial response at 400 mg/day. Obtaining the maximum response to imatinib can require 3–12 months of therapy, with a median of 6 months.

At present, it is advised that imatinib therapy should be continued unless there is disease progression, drug intolerance, or patient non-compliance. In the event of surgery, the drug is stopped the day before surgery and resumed when oral medications are tolerated.

## Side Effects

Overall, imatinib is well tolerated, and only 5% of patients undergo interruption of therapy because of toxicity. Toxicity is usually controllable and includes periorbital edema, rash, diarrhea, nausea, abdominal pain, and fatigue.

Side effects are usually mild to moderate and transient, and can be managed without dose interruption. There is about a 5% risk of tumor hemorrhage. Neutropenia and liver toxicity are uncommon, but blood tests must be monitored routinely.

## Evaluation of Response to Therapy

CT is the preferred method in evaluating the response to tyrosine kinase inhibitor (TKI) therapy, unless a very short-term follow-up of within 1–2 weeks is needed (e.g., to make a surgical decision for those with marginally resectable tumors). It is important to realize that response to molecular therapy in GIST is not always accompanied by a reduction in tumor diameter. The appearance of a new nodule in the context of a hypodense lesion, which represents early progression of disease (Fig. 18.2), is also not interpreted properly if only external dimensions are considered. GIST treated

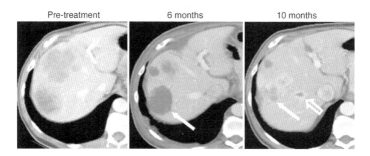

FIGURE 18.2. Acquired resistance to imatinib. The patient had multiple liver metastases and initially had a response to imatinib mesylate. Note the decrease in contrast enhancement at 6 months by CT scan. The presence of a small nodule (*solid arrow*) represents residual tumor. While still on imatinib, the patient progressed at 10 months (*solid arrow*) and the tumor extended down the right hepatic vein (*open arrow*) (Reprinted from Van der Zwan and DeMatteo, 2005. With kind permission of Lippincott Williams & Wilkins).

with TKI can increase in volume as a consequence of myxoid degeneration of the tumoral content, intratumoral hemorrhage or edema of the lesion. A better marker of treatment response is tumor density; the tumoral mass often changes in appearance from hypervascular to hypoattenuating and homogeneous. In some cases, the initial density of the hepatic lesions can be similar to that of normal hepatic parenchyma, making them invisible on portal venous phases. Thus, non-contrast and arterial phase images are indicated. Responding liver lesions that decrease in density can become cystic and can be mistakenly interpreted as new lesions. Histologically, the cystic lesions contain hyaline degeneration and residual KIT-positive cells. The optimal criteria for the evaluation of the tumor response should include size, density and metabolic activity. When it is necessary to determine the early response to TKI, an 18-FDG PETscan can be performed. PET scan can demonstrate a response to TKI within a few days, while CT scan requires several weeks of treatment. Overall, however, nearly all patients can be managed by CT scan alone.

## Prediction of Response Based on Mutation Status

The therapeutic response of GIST to imatinib appears to be related to the mutation status of *KIT* and *PDGFRα*. Typically, GISTs with exon 11 mutation have the highest chance of response to imatinib, while wild-type or exon 9 mutated GISTs have a lower chance. Little is known regarding the effect of imatinib on KIT-negative GIST, but there appears to be clinical benefit. Not all the *PDGFRα* activating mutations are biologically equivalent, as some are characterized by relative insensitivity to imatinib while others confer sensitivity. Because specific *PDGFRα* mutation analysis is typically not carried out in GIST, patients with advanced tumors that appear histologically compatible with GIST should not be denied a trial of imatinib if their tumor is KIT negative.

## Clinical Applications

The efficacy of TKI therapy in advanced GIST has prompted interest in its use in the adjuvant setting for patients with primary disease at high risk of recurrence postoperatively, or as preoperative or induction therapy in patients with localized unresectable (or borderline resectable) tumors. Trials are ongoing to evaluate the role of molecular targeted therapy in these settings.

Neoadjuvant therapy is particularly attractive for patients with large or poorly placed tumors that are marginally resectable or tumors that would require extensive sacrifice of normal tissue. For instance, neoadjuvant imatinib may convert the resection of a rectal GIST from an abdominoperineal resection to a low anterior resection. While it is postulated that surgical resection might become a feasible option after imatinib therapy in some patients who present with initially unresectable disease, this concept has not been evaluated rigorously. Thus, neoadjuvant therapy should be tested in clinical trials. Neoadjuvant therapy used for patients with resectable disease with the goal of eradicating potential subclinical metastatic disease is another experimental approach.

## Adjuvant Therapy

At present, adjuvant therapy with imatinib is investigational, and should not be employed in the routine postoperative treatment of patients after complete resection of high-risk tumors outside of clinical trials. Various studies are ongoing to evaluate the activity of imatinib as an adjuvant following the complete resection of a primary GIST. The American College of Surgeons Oncology Group (ACOSOG) is leading a Phase II intergroup trial testing the value of adjuvant imatinib at a dose of 400 mg/day for 12 months after complete macroscopic surgical resection in patients with high-risk primary GIST. High risk is defined as a tumor size $\geq 10$ cm, intraperitoneal tumor rupture or hemorrhage, or multifocal tumors. Survival in this study will be compared with that of historical controls. The initial data from this trial have shown that imatinib is well tolerated in the adjuvant setting, and 83% of the patients completed the 12 months of imatinib therapy. In addition, a randomized, double-blinded Phase III ACOSOG intergroup trial is open for patients with tumors measuring at least 3 cm. Patients receive imatinib (400 mg/day) or placebo for 1 year after undergoing complete resection of their primary GIST. Patients assigned to the placebo arm will cross over to imatinib therapy in the event of tumor recurrence. The primary endpoint is recurrence-free survival between the two arms. EORTC is also conducting a trial to determine the benefit of adjuvant imatinib in moderate to high-risk patients.

## Outcome

No prospective data exist regarding the outcome of patients with primary GIST and existing data are from the pre-imatinib era. Five-year survival rates range from 50% to 80%. In one report, median disease-specific survival was 60 months with primary disease, 19 months with metastatic disease, and 12 months with local recurrence. Complete resection is accomplished in approximately 85% of patients with primary disease. The availability of TKI therapy will undoubtedly improve these results.

## Follow-Up

There is no standard postoperative follow-up in patients who undergo surgical resection of a primary GIST. In general, there is no proof that earlier detection of recurrent GIST improves survival. However, because there is now an effective treatment for patients with recurrent or metastatic disease, it appears reasonable to perform routine postoperative surveillance. The National Comprehensive Cancer Network (NCCN) consensus panel recommends CT scans of the abdomen and pelvis with intravenous contrast every 3–6 months during the first 3–5 years and possibly yearly thereafter. In metastatic disease, scans are undertaken typically every 3–4 months to assess response and monitor for resistance.

## Recurrence

The majority of patients will experience tumor recurrence despite undergoing complete resection of their primary tumor. The median time to recurrence after surgery is reported to range from 18–24 months. The first site of recurrence of GIST is usually within the abdomen and involves the peritoneum and/or the liver. At the time of disease recurrence, approximately two-thirds of patients have liver involvement and half have peritoneal disease. Extraabdominal metastases (e.g., lung or bone) may develop later in the course of the disease. Typically, peritoneal disease is found to be more extensive than what is indicated on preoperative imaging. Removal of peritoneal metastases was usually followed by subsequent recurrence in the era before TKI therapy. Liver metastases from GIST are usually multifocal. Surgery alone has limited efficacy in recurrent GIST. Recurrent GISTs are now treated with TKI treatment and the median survival exceeds 5 years. Recurrence usually culminated in death within 18 months previously.

## TKI Resistance

Resistance to imatinib or sunitinib occurs in patients who have had an initial therapeutic response. In patients with imatinib-resistant disease, KIT activation still plays a functional role in the majority of tumors. *KIT* exon 9 mutations, D824V substitutions in *PDGFRα* or the presence of a wild-type *KIT* gene are the most frequent causes of **primary resistance**, that can be observed in about 15% of cases and is defined as disease progression within the first 6 months of therapy with imatinib. This type of progression is usually multifocal. In the case of **secondary resistance**, disease progression occurs after the first 6 months of therapy with imatinib.

Secondary resistance may be partial (the presence of a nodule of progressive disease in the context of one or a limited number of secondary lesions) or multifocal and diffuse. Selection of clones with secondary *KIT* or *PDGFRα* mutations appears to be the most common mechanism of imatinib resistance.

## Management of Tumor Progression

Disease progression is determined with radiologic imaging. In the case of primary resistance, tumor pathology should be re-evaluated to confirm the diagnosis of GIST. Disease progression can be focal or multifocal. In patients who develop focal resistance to imatinib (i.e., one specific tumor begins to grow again), surgery should be considered, although the benefit of this approach is unknown. Alternatives to surgery for residual GIST liver metastases include radiofrequency ablation (RFA) and hepatic artery embolization. It is important to continue the therapy with imatinib, the dosage of which can be increased to 800 mg/day, if tolerated, with the purpose to prevent or delay the onset of further resistant clones. Dose escalation may also temporize multifocal disease progression in some patients. There is general agreement that multifocal resistance to imatinib should be treated with another targeted agent such as sunitinib. Sunitinib is a multi-kinase inhibitor acting on the KIT, PDGFR, VEGFR, RET and *fms*-related tyrosine kinase 3 (FLT3) receptors. In the initial clinical studies, sunitinib produced a partial response in 10% of patients and stable disease in about 60% with disease progression after imatinib. Sunitinib has more side effects than imatinib and include frequently fatigue (34%), diarrhea (29%), skin discoloration (25%), nausea (24%), anorexia (19%), stomatitis (16%), vomit (16%), cutaneous rash (13%) and anemia (12%). The efficacy of sunitinib raises the question of whether it may be more effective than imatinib as a first line agent. In particular, since sunitinib is more likely than imatinib to work in exon 9 mutation, consideration should be given to using it primarily in those patients.

## Other Agents

A variety of other agents are being developed and tested for GIST. Everolimus (RAD001) is an inhibitor of mTOR. Other drugs include PKC412 (inhibits pKC, VEGFR, PDGFR, KIT isoenzymes), BMS 354825 (dasatinib – inhibits BCR-ABL, Src, KIT, PDGFR), AMG706 (inhibits KIT, PDGFR, VEGF, RET), and bevacizumab.

# Selected Readings

Antonescu CR, Besmer P, Guo T et al. (2005) Acquired resistance to imatinib in gastrointestinal stromal tumor occurs through secondary gene mutation. Clin Cancer Res 11:4182–4190

Antonescu CR, Viale A, Sarran L et al. (2004) Gene expression in gastrointestinal stromal tumors is distinguished by KIT genotype and anatomic site. Clin Cancer Res 10:3282–3290

Debiec-Rychter M, Cools J, Dumez H et al. (2005) Mechanisms of resistance to imatinib mesylate in gastrointestinal stromal tumors and activity of the PKC412 inhibitor against imatinib-resistant mutants. Gastroenterology 128:270–279

DeMatteo RP, Lewis JJ, Leung D et al. (2000) Two hundred gastrointestinal stromal tumors: recurrence patterns and prognostic factors for survival. Ann Surg 231:51–58

Heinrich MC, Corless CL, Demetri GD et al. (2003) Kinase mutations and imatinib response in patients with metastatic gastrointestinal stromal tumor. J Clin Oncol 21(23):4342–4349

Heinrich MC, Corless CL, Duensing A et al. (2003) PDGFRA activating mutations in gastrointestinal stromal tumors. Science 299:708–710

Maki RG, Fletcher JA, Heinrich MC et al. (2005) SU11248, a multi-targeted tyrosine kinase inhibitor, can overcome imatinib (IM) resistance caused by diverse genomic mechanisms in patients (pts) with metastatic gastrointestinal stromal tumor (GIST). Proc Am Soc Clin Oncol 23:9011 (abstract)

Miettinen M, El-Rifai W, Sobin LH, Lasota J (2002) Evaluation of malignancy and prognosis of gastrointestinal stromal tumors: a review. Human Pathol 33:478–483

Van der Zwan SM, DeMatteo RP (2005) Gastrointestinal stromal tumor: 5 years later. Cancer 104:1781–1788

Verweij J, Casali PG, Zalcberg J et al. (2004) Progression-free survival in gastrointestinal stromal tumours with high-dose imatinib: randomised trial. Lancet 364:1127–1134

# 19
# Gastric Lymphoma

**John H. Donohue**

## Pearls and Pitfalls

- With rare exceptions, gastric lymphoma is no longer a surgical disease.
- Most low-grade MALT lymphomas respond completely to *H. pylori* eradication.
- MALT lymphomas require months to regress completely after successful *H. pylori* eradication. While monoclonal B lymphocytes may persist for years, clinical relapse is unusual without recurrent *H. pylori* infection.
- For gastric MALT lymphomas, resistance to *H. pylori* treatment can be predicted by genetic mutations, more extensive disease, and the presence of high-grade cytopathology.
- Unresponsive gastric MALT lymphomas can usually be salvaged with radiation therapy, cyclophosphamide, rituximab, or CVP ± rituximab chemotherapy.
- Regardless of treatment type, the 10-year survival of patients with gastric MALT lymphomas is ≥90% with 10-year event-free survivals of about 70%.
- High-grade gastric lymphomas (diffuse B-cell lymphomas comprise the majority) should be treated with combination chemotherapy (most often CHOP) ± radiation therapy.
- Operative therapy of gastric lymphoma is generally now restricted to patients with localized, residual, high-grade neoplasms after nonsurgical therapy or complications of the lymphoma (hemorrhage, obstruction, and perforation).

K.I. Bland et al. (eds.), *Surgery of the Esophagus and Stomach*, DOI: 10.1007/978-1-84996-438-8_19,
© Springer-Verlag London Limited 2011

- Survival with high-grade gastric lymphomas is less than for MALT lymphomas and is stage-dependent (5-year overall survival: stage IE ~ 90%, Stage IIE ~70–80%, Stage IV ~ 50%).

## Basic Science

More than 90% of patients with gastric lymphoma have a Helicobacter pylori (*H. pylori*) infection. Despite the absence of lymphoid tissue in the stomach wall, a chronic *H. pylori* infection may cause a gastric mucosa-associated lymphoid tissue (MALT) lymphoma. Gastric MALTs contain a monoclonal population of B-cells, the proliferation of which is controlled by a small number of T-lymphocytes whose stimulation is dependent on the presence of the specific infecting strain of *H. pylori*.

In most gastric MALT lymphomas, *H. pylori* eradication results in cessation of the B-cell proliferation and eventual resolution of the lymphoma infiltrate. The presence of specific chromosomal translocation and other genetic changes (see Fig. 19.1) results in most failures of gastric MALT lymphomas to respond to *H. pylori* therapy and the progression of a MALT lymphoma to a high-grade gastric lymphoma. It is unknown how often pure high-grade lymphomas arise from a MALT lymphoma versus occurring *de novo*.

# Clinical Presentation

Epigastric pain or dyspepsia is the most common symptom of gastric lymphoma. Clinically significant hemorrhage occurs in only a small number of patients. Advanced stage, high-grade gastric lymphoma may produce constitutional complaints of weight loss, fatigue, fevers, and night sweats (B symptoms) and/or an epigastric mass. Peripheral adenopathy is not present with primary lymphomas of the stomach. The absence of specific symptoms and signs make a clinical

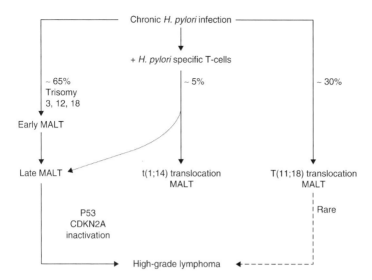

FIGURE 19.1. Progression of gastric MALT lymphomas. Gastric MALT lymphomas occur with chronic *H. pylori* infection and the presence of *H. pylori* specific T-cells. B-cell proliferation becomes less dependent on *H. pylori* antigenic stimulation from the top to the bottom (late MALT and most t(1;14) and t(11;18) translocation MALTs are unresponsive to *H. pylori* therapy) (Adapted from Isaacson and Du 2004. Copyright 2004. With permission from Macmillan).

diagnosis of gastric lymphoma virtually impossible without a tissue biopsy.

# Diagnosis

Upper gastrointestinal endoscopy (EGD) with biopsy is the diagnostic test of choice. Most gastric lymphomas infiltrate the stomach wall diffusely, similar to a diffuse gastric adeno-carcinoma, but discrete masses, ulcerated tumors, and even polypoid lesions can all occur. The gastric biopsies should be evaluated for both the histologic type of lymphoma and the presence of *H. pylori*. Endoscopic ultrasonography (EUS)

TABLE 19.1. Musshoff staging system for gastric lymphomas.

| Stage | Disease extent |
|-------|----------------|
| IE | Stomach only |
| IIEi | Perigastric nodes |
| IIEii | Para-aortic nodes |
| III | Spleen |
| IV | Distant site(s) (usually bone marrow) |

*E: extranodal lymphoma.*

allows determination of both the depth of primary tumor invasion and the presence of nodal involvement (which can be documented with fine-needle aspiration). Findings of more extensive disease are especially helpful in MALT lymphomas, because they indicate the likely need for more treatment than just *H. pylori* eradication.

Once lymphoma of the stomach is diagnosed with a biopsy, computed tomography (CT) of the abdomen should be obtained for staging. A lymphangiogram is not indicated. Most experts recommend a thorough head and neck evaluation to rule out involvement of the MALT tissues in Waldeyer's ring. A chest radiograph and bone marrow biopsy complete the staging process. The Musshoff modification of the Ann Arbor lymphoma staging system (see Table 19.1) is used for gastric lymphomas.

## Treatment

Therapy for gastric lymphoma depends on the histology and is normally divided into treatment for low-grade gastric MALT lymphoma and high-grade lymphomas of the stomach. Because the vast majority of high-grade gastric lymphomas are diffuse B-cell types, only the treatment for this form of lymphoma will be discussed. T-cell lymphomas and other variants of B-cell lymphoma are quite uncommon, and their specific management will not be covered in this chapter.

*MALT lymphomas*: More than 90% of gastric MALT lymphoma patients are infected by *H. pylori*. *H. pylori* eradication is undertaken with a 2-week course of antibiotics, usually clarithromycin and amoxicillin (or metronidazole), plus a proton pump inhibitor to suppress acid secretion. Bismuth compounds are used less commonly than in the past. Confirmation of successful *H. pylori* elimination should be obtained with repeat gastric biopsies or a breath test. Repeat treatment with different antibiotics is indicated when the *H. pylori* infection is resistant to the first-line therapy.

The histologic resolution of MALT lymphomas requires an average of 3–6 months but on occasion may take up to 28 months. Repeat EGD with biopsies and EUS should be performed every three months until there is complete resolution (CR) of the neoplasm on imaging and microscopic evaluation. Endoscopic surveillance is continued after this every 6–12 months, because monoclonal B-cells are still present in ≥25% of MALT lymphoma patients after CR. After a histologic CR, less than 20% of patients will have a microscopic histologic relapse, and mostly when a monoclonal pattern of B-cells persists. Surprisingly, these microscopic recrudescences of disease normally resolve with a watch-and-wait approach. Macroscopic recurrent lymphoma in a MALT lymphoma patient with a CR is rare, unless there is recurrent *H. pylori* infection.

In the 10% of patients with gastric MALT lymphoma who are negative for *H. pylori* or those infected with *H. pylori* that does not respond to bacterial eradication therapy, other methods of treatment are indicated (see Fig. 19.2). Patients with a t(11;18) translocation (approximately 30% of all MALT tumors), including those with an *H. pylori* infection, are often resistant to treatment that eradicates *H. pylori*. Recent data suggest resistance of this genotype to therapy with oral cyclophosphamide agents. The MALT lymphomas that contain a component of high-grade lymphomas are also more likely not to respond to *H. pylori* eradication alone. Second-line therapies for resistant MALT lymphomas include

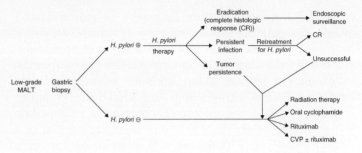

FIGURE 19.2. Treatment of low-grade gastric MALT lymphomas.

radiation therapy (30 gray [Gy] in 150 cGy fractions over 4 weeks), oral cyclophosphamide (100 mg/day for 6–12 months), monoclonal anti-CD20 antibody (rituximab 375 mg/m$^2$ weekly x4) combination chemotherapy (cyclophosphamide, vincristine, and prednisone [CVP often with rituximab]) or combinations of these treatments. Some lymphomas with a component of high-grade lymphoma coexisting with a low-grade gastric MALT lymphoma will respond completely to *H. pylori* therapy, but there is greater probability that combination chemotherapy will be needed to produce a complete response. At least one recent report has noted a higher likelihood of eradicating residual microscopic, monoclonal B-cell proliferation after combined chemotherapy and radiation therapy for MALT, mixed MALT-high-grade, and pure high-grade gastric lymphomas.

*High-grade gastric lymphomas*: Patients with high-grade lymphomas require treatment with combination chemotherapy. Bulky disease, especially when residual disease persists, will benefit from the addition of radiation therapy. High-grade gastric lymphomas have diffuse, large-cell characteristics and respond best to R-CHOP chemotherapy (rituximab, cyclophosphamide, doxorubicin, vincristine, and prednisone). Rarer types of B-cell lymphomas and T-cell lymphomas should be treated in a fashion similar to the same histology at other primary sites. The management algorithm for high-grade, diffuse, large-cell gastric lymphoma is outlined in Fig. 19.3.

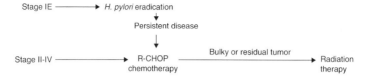

FIGURE 19.3. Management of gastric high-grade lymphomas.

# Outcome

Several randomized and nonrandomized prospective trials comparing operative treatment for clinical stage IE and IIE disease patients (some with and others without adjuvant therapy) versus nonsurgical therapy have shown patient survival to be the same or better for the nonsurgical treatment groups. In all studies, the frequency and severity of complications of the surgical group has been greater than for nonsurgical patients. These studies have hastened the move to defer operative intervention in patients with gastric lymphoma unless the patient has a rare complication from nonsurgical treatment or localized persistent lymphoma. Despite concerns about perforation and hemorrhage during the chemotherapy, these complications are rare in patients with gastric lymphoma. Operative therapy for gastric lymphoma is now the exception rather than the normal treatment for any stage of gastric lymphoma.

In clinical stage IE MALT lymphoma, 10-year survival is generally > 90% with *H. pylori* treatment or secondary therapies, when indicated. Treatment outcomes are similar for clinical stage IE high-grade gastric lymphomas. Mixed MALT high-grade and high-grade stage IIE gastric lymphomas have approximately a 70–80% chance of 5-year survival with nonsurgical therapy. Patients with stage IV gastric lymphoma have a 5-year survival of about 50%. Patients with T-cell or rarer types of high-grade B-cell lymphoma of the stomach generally have poorer outcomes than patients with diffuse large-cell lymphomas.

# Selected Readings

Alpen B, Kuse R, Parwaresch R et al. (2004) Ongoing monoclonal B-cell proliferation is not common in gastric B-cell lymphoma after combined radiochemotherapy. J Clin Oncol 22:3039–3045

Avilés A, Nambo J, Neri N et al. (2004) The role of surgery in primary gastric lymphoma: results of a controlled clinical trial. Ann Surg 240:44–50

Alvilés A, Nambo MJ, Neri N et al. (2005) Mucosa-associated lymphoid tissue (MALT) lymphoma of the stomach: results of a controlled clinical trial. Med Oncol 22:57–62

Chen LT, Lin JT, Tai JJ et al. (2005) Long-term results of anti-Helicobacter pylori therapy in early-stage gastric high-grade transformed MALT lymphoma. J Natl Cancer Inst 97:1345–1353

Isaacson PG, Du M-Q (2004) MALT lymphoma: from morphology to molecules. Nat Rev 4:644–653

Koch P, Probst A, Berdel WE et al. (2005) Treatment results in localized primary gastric lymphoma: data of patients registered within the German Multicenter Study (GIT NHL 02/96). J Clin Oncol 23:7050–7059

Lévy M, Copie-Bergman C, Gameiro C et al. (2005) Prognostic value of translocation t (11;18) in tumoral response of low-grade gastric lymphoma of mucosa-associated lymphoid tissue type to oral chemotherapy. J Clin Oncol 23:5061–5066

Martinelli G, Laszlo D, Ferreri AJM et al. (2005) Clinical activity of rituximab in gastric marginal zone non Hodgkin's lymphoma resistant to or not eligible for anti-Helicobacter pylori therapy. J Clin Oncol 23:1979–1983

Nakamura S, Matsumoto T, Suekane H et al. (2005) Long-term clinical outcome of *Helicobacter pylori* eradication for gastric mucosa-associated lymphoid tissue lymphoma with reference to second-line treatment. Cancer 104:532–540

Wündisch T, Thiede C, Morgner A et al. (2005) Long-term follow-up of gastric MALT lymphoma after Helicobacter pylori eradication. J Clin Oncol 23:8018–8024

Yoon SS, Coit DG, Portlock CS, Karpeh MS (2004) The diminishing role of surgery in the treatment of gastric lymphoma. Ann Surg 240:28–37

# Part IV
# Gastrointestinal Bleeding

# 20
# Upper Gastrointestinal Hemorrhage: Diagnosis and Treatment

**Joaquim Gama-Rodrigues, Igor Proscurshim, and Carlos Eduardo Jacob**

## Pearls and Pitfalls

- Patients with acute upper GI bleeding require aggressive resuscitation.
- Patients with recent or active bleeding need a large bore, intravenous line during the initial evaluation.
- ALWAYS attempt endoscopic control for upper GI bleeding.
- In elderly patients, the hematocrit should be kept above 30%, while in young healthy patients, above 20%.
- Patients that require monitoring should be admitted to an intensive care unit.
- Peptic ulcer is the most common cause of upper GI bleeding.
- Signs of chronic liver disease should be sought.
- All patients with suspected or proven upper GI bleeding require a panendoscopy with the purpose of diagnosis and potentially therapy.
- For occult GI bleeding, diagnosis of the site and cause may require repeated endoscopic examinations, enteroscopy, video capsule endoscopy, barium contrast series, enteroclysis, angiography, and RBC-tagged radionucleotide scan.

K.I. Bland et al. (eds.), *Surgery of the Esophagus and Stomach*, DOI: 10.1007/978-1-84996-438-8_20, © Springer-Verlag London Limited 2011

- Aggressive therapy with proton pump inhibitors combined with antibiotics to eradicate *Helicobacter pylori* infection may be effective in controlling peptic ulcer bleeding.
- Hemodynamically unstable patients or those with ongoing bleeding should be considered for immediate operative intervention.
- Gastric resection or vagotomy has a relatively high rate of morbidity and rebleeding.
- Try to avoid operative intervention in patients who are candidates for liver transplantation.

# Upper Gastrointestinal Hemorrhage – Diagnosis and Treatment

Upper gastrointestinal (GI) bleeding is a common condition that obligates a high morbidity and health care burden. The most common causes of upper gastrointestinal bleeding are peptic ulcer, gastroesophageal varices, arteriovenous malformations, Mallory-Weiss tears, erosive gastritis, and neoplasms, both benign and malignant. Patients with upper GI bleeding may present with hematemesis, hematochezia, hypotension-related symptoms, and melena or with a positive screening fecal occult blood test (FOBT) or chronic iron-deficient anemia with no obvious source of blood loss. Esophagogastroduodenoscopy (EGD) is the diagnostic examination of choice for upper GI bleeding and should be performed in most all suspected cases. Urgency of the initial management is based on the amount and acuteness of the blood loss. Patients who are hemodynamically unstable or have active bleeding need to be hospitalized and managed aggressively, while selected patients who are hemodynamically stable with no evidence of active bleeding may be managed in an outpatient setting. Upper GI bleeding can be acute requiring immediate intervention, occult and remain subclinical for years, or obscure which is not readily diagnosed, all of which may require extensive investigation.

# Acute Upper GI Bleeding

The most common cause of acute upper GI bleeding are peptic ulcers, encompassing about 60% of all patients, followed by erosive gastritis (15%), and variceal bleeding (6%). Patients with acute upper GI bleeding usually present with signs of hemodynamic instability, such as dizziness, light-headedness, weakness, pallor, palpitations, tachycardia, orthostatic hypotension, shock, and even cardiopulmonary arrest. Bleeding in these patients is usually evidenced by hematemesis, melena, or even hematochezia which may be found in over 14% of patients with upper GI bleeding.

## Initial Assessment

Patients with suspected acute upper GI bleeding should be assessed rapidly and stabilized. Unstable patients and stable patients with active or recent bleeding need a large-bore intravenous (IV) catheter placed during the initial workup. Blood loss needs to be estimated and the bleeding localized. If the patient is unstable, immediate resuscitation should be started.

*Resuscitation*: The unstable patient with active or recent bleeding needs to be managed aggressively. Airway, breathing, and circulation (the ABCs) should be assessed immediately and appropriate interventions instituted when necessary. Infusion of fluid with 0.9% normal saline or Ringer's lactate (RL) through large-bore IV lines or a central line should be started and blood transfused as needed to maintain tissue perfusion; in elderly patients, the hematocrit should be kept above 30%, while in young, healthy patients, the target hematocrit should be above 20%. A urinary catheter may be needed to monitor urine output, and any coagulopathy should be sought and corrected. These patients should be monitored in an intensive care unit. When the patient stabilizes, an emergent evaluation should be undertaken; however, if the patient remains unstable, the patient should undergo emergent EGD and/or operative intervention, depending on the severity of bleeding and knowledge of the site of bleeding.

## Emergent Evaluation

*Patient history*: Medical history should include investigation of prior episodes of upper gastrointestinal bleeding (ulcers or varices), liver disease, intestinal polyps or cancer, and blood transfusions. Alcohol abuse and illicit drug use should also be investigated. A careful history of medication use must be taken, including use of aspirin, nonsteroidal anti-inflammatory drugs (NSAIDs), and anticoagulation drugs (warfarin, heparin). Symptoms such as abdominal pain, nausea, vomiting, hematemesis, early satiety, anorexia, and weight loss should be sought. A cardiac history is important to determine the threshold for blood transfusion.

*Physical examination*: Careful attention should be paid to signs of chronic liver disease, such as jaundice, caput medusae, spider telangiectasia, and/or ascites. Physical examination should include a digital rectal examination and an NG tube aspiration. If the NG aspirate is bloody and/or if a non-gastric upper GI source is suspected, an upper GI endoscopy is recommended; if, however, the aspirate is bilious or clear and there is no clinical evidence for upper GI bleeding, a colonoscopy is indicated.

*Initial work-up*: Initial blood work should include a complete blood count, liver and renal function tests, coagulation parameters (PT/INR, PTT), and typing and crossmatching. Chest and abdominal x-rays are also needed (these tests may indicate perforation or aspiration), and an ECG is warranted, for patients with cardiovascular risk factors. Early risk stratification into high risk or low risk for re-bleeding or mortality using a validated risk scale, such as the Rockall or Baylor risk scales, may be beneficial for the health care team (Table 20.1). If there is a high risk of rebleeding or mortality, the patient should be hospitalized, investigated, and treated. Patients that have a low risk can be managed in an outpatient setting.

## Emergent Management

*Detection and diagnosis*: All patients with suspected upper GI bleeding probably require an endoscopy. In the emergent

TABLE 20.1.  Risk factors for upper GI bleeding.

| Risk factors for upper GI bleeding |
| --- |
| Older age (>60 years) |
| Severe comorbidity |
| Active bleeding |
| Hypotension or shock |
| Red blood cell transfusion ≥6 units |
| Inpatient status at time of bleed |
| Severe coagulopathy |
| High risk endoscopic stigmata |

setting, a gentle gastric lavage with warm, 0.9% saline through the NG tube should be performed prior to endoscopy to remove blood and food particulate matter. This irrigation permits better visualization of the upper GI tract and decreases the chance of massive aspiration. EGD not only detects the location of the bleeding but may also diagnose the underlying cause and control the bleeding. If the EGD is negative and an upper GI source is still suspected, a red blood cell-tagged radionucleotide scan should be considered. Barium studies are not indicated in acute upper GI bleeding, because the contrast interferes with endoscopy and potential operation.

*Emergent treatment*: Variceal bleeding can be treated endoscopically with band-ligation or injection sclerotherapy, which can be used concomitantly with octreotide, somatostatin, or glypressin (octreotide: 50 mg IV bolus followed by 50 mg per 8–24 h; Somatostatin: 250–500 mg IV bolus followed by 250–500 mg per hour; glypressin: 2 mg bolus IV followed by 1 mg per hour). Endoscopic sclerotherapy combined with this drug therapy is better than sclerotherapy alone.

Endoscopic hemostasis should always be attempted in patients with non-variceal bleeding. Hemostasis can be achieved either by injection sclerotherapy, electrocoagulation, heater probes, or laser therapy. Concomitant drug therapy with high-dose, proton-pump inhibitors (PPI; IV bolus followed by continuous infusion) improves outcome, decreases rebleeding rate, and decreases hospital stay. If endoscopic control fails, radiologic intervention, balloon tamponade, and operative intervention with or without intra-operative endoscopy should be considered (Fig. 20.1).

## Occult Upper GI Bleeding

Upper GI bleeding is not always overt or associated with the classic signs of hematemesis and melena but may present as a chronic iron-deficiency anemia or a positive FOBT without any visible bleeding. These patients should stimulate a high degree of suspicion and should be investigated thoroughly for the source of blood loss. A detailed medical history is fundamental and includes investigation of liver disease, intestinal polyps or cancer, blood transfusions, alcohol abuse, and illicit drug use. As with acute bleeding, a careful history of medication use including over-the-counter medication is imperative. Symptoms such as abdominal pain, nausea, vomiting, early satiety, anorexia, or weight loss should be sought and careful attention paid to signs of chronic liver disease.

Colonoscopy and EGD are the first investigations for occult bleeding; however, in about 50% of patients, the source of the bleeding is not found. If the EGD shows the underlying cause, medical, endoscopic, or operative therapy are instituted. If both colonoscopy and EGD are negative, further immediate investigation may not be necessary especially in younger patients; however, if positive FOBTs or iron-deficiency persists, further investigation is necessary as described for obscure GI bleeding (Fig. 20.2).

## Obscure Upper GI Bleeding

Obscure upper GI bleeding is defined as recurrent overt or occult bleeding after an initial negative endoscopic examination. If the bleeding is overt with evidence of ongoing blood loss, the patient should be evaluated as an acute upper GI bleed; in these patients, a RBC-tagged radionucleotide scan is

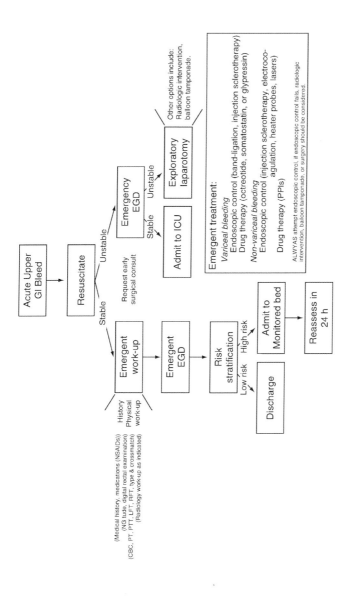

FIGURE 20.1. Acute upper GI bleeding algorithm.

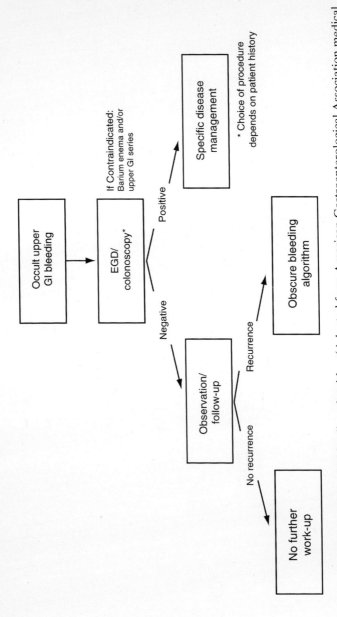

FIGURE 20.2. Occult upper GI bleeding algorithm (Adapted from American Gastroenterological Association medical position statement, 2000. With permission).

recommended as part of the diagnostic work-up. For the remaining patients, a repeat endoscopy with enteroscopy is recommended; if negative, these endoscopic modalities should be followed by enteroclysis or small bowel series, and possibly angiography. Finally, if the bleeding persists and diagnostic exams are inconclusive, consideration should be given to exploratory operation with intraoperative enteroscopy.

## Diagnostic Modalities

### Endoscopy

*Conventional EGD*: All patients with suspected upper GI bleeding and without any contraindications should eventually undergo an EGD. Gentle gastric lavage with 0.9% normal saline may be needed to remove blood and particulate matter to improve visualization. Erythromycin given intravenously (250 mg IV bolus or 3 mg/kg IV over 20–30 min) 20–90 min before endoscopy improves visibility and decreases endoscopy time. The EGD can detect and diagnose most sources of upper GI bleeding and allows tissue biopsy for pathologic examination and hemostasis. Numerous techniques are available for control of bleeding, including electrocautery, heat probe, laser therapy, band ligation, clip placement, injection sclerotherapy, and injection of cryanoacrylic glue.

*Enteroscopy*: Visualization of the entire small bowel mucosa remains a challenge to endoscopists. Push enteroscopy, in which an enteroscope is pushed beyond the ligament of Trietz, is the standard approach. This technique has a diagnostic yield of about 60%, because a significant proportion of lesions detected by the enteroscope are within reach of the endoscope. A "second look" EGD may be recommended before an enteroscopy is planned. Newer extended techniques such as double balloon enteroscopy show promising results but remain to be validated. These techniques often do not permit therapeutic intervention and may not provide reliable information of distance from the ligament of Treitz.

*Video capsule endoscopy*: Video capsule endoscopy is a recent, nearly non-invasive technique in which a small capsule (11 mm with camera, lens, and transmitter) is ingested orally by the patient and transmits images to a receiver. This technique can diagnose a site of bleeding in over 50% of patients with obscure bleeding using negative push endoscopy. Its drawbacks are that it is inefficient in the esophagus and stomach and does not permit tissue sampling, intervention, or clear identification of where exactly in the jejunoileum the abnormality is located. It is, however, an excellent diagnostic tool that should be considered, especially in patients with obscure bleeding in whom an exploratory operation is the next step. On rare occasions, the capsule may become entrapped and require operative removal and therefore should not be used in patients with suspected strictures or known extensive adhesions.

## Radiology

*Barium contrast series*: In the emergency setting, barium studies are contraindicated, because barium interferes with endoscopic and operative visualization. In the elective setting and especially in the investigation of obscure bleeding, a barium contrast series has a high diagnostic yield for small bowel bleeds secondary to a mass lesion and can be used before push enteroscopy in high-risk patients or after a negative push enteroscopy.

*Enteroclysis*: Enteroclysis is a double-contrast study performed by passing a tube into the proximal small bowel and injecting barium, methylcellulose, and air often in conjunction with intravenous glucagon. This technique has a greater diagnostic yield than conventional imaging because of its increased resolution and lack of an overlapping, barium-filled stomach, but due to patient discomfort, its use is limited. One should consider this technique selectively.

*Angiography*: Angiography is usually reserved for bleeding that either was not detected by conventional strategies or in patients in whom other treatments have failed. Angiography can detect a bleeding rate of greater than 0.5 ml/min; active bleeding is seen as extravasation of contrast into the lumen of the bowel, but angiography will also show abnormal vessels or vascular blushes even in the absence of active bleeding. Angiography permits selective infusion of a vasoconstrictor, such as vasopressin and/or embolization with gelfoam, polyvinyl alcohol, or a solid blocking material. In hemorrhagic gastritis, selective arterial injection of vasopressin should be attempted if medical treatment fails. Angiography with selective intraarterial embolization is the treatment of choice for hemobilia and remains the best method for diagnosis.

*Radionucleotide scans*: Radionucleotide scans with either Technetium pertechnate-labeled autologous red blood cells or Technetium sulfur colloid can detect bleeding at a rate of 0.1–0.4 ml/min. This technique is extremely sensitive but is less specific than an endoscopy or arteriography and often only localizes the site of bleeding to an area of abdomen. Confirmation with either an arteriography or endoscopy may be necessary.

*Operative exploration/intraoperative enteroscopy*: Celiotomy for intraoperative endoscopy is the last resort for diagnosing and/or treating acute GI bleeding not detected or amenable to other interventions and for diagnosing thoroughly investigated obscure, recurrent GI bleeding requiring multiple transfusions (Fig. 20.3). Intraoperative enteroscopy is usually best performed by making a mid small bowel enterotomy and examining the bowel lumen proximally and distally during a gradual controlled insertion of the endoscope rather than after telescoping the bowel over the endoscope and examining the mucosa while removing the tube. Passing the endoscope into the small bowel either by mouth or per anus is much less effective and may not allow visualization of the entire jejunoileum.

# Management of Specific Causes of Upper GI Bleeding

## Peptic Ulcers

Peptic ulcers are the most frequent cause of upper GI bleeding. Aggressive medical therapy with PPIs combined with endoscopic, interventional, therapeutic techniques is

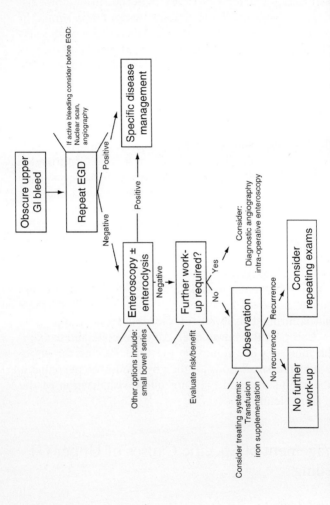

FIGURE 20.3.  Obscure upper GI bleeding algorithm (Adapted from American Gastroenterological Association medical position statement, 2000. With permission).

extremely effective in controlling the acute phase of peptic ulcer bleeding. The success of this approach may create a dilemma for the surgeon in deciding whether or not to continue with a non-operative approach or to submit the patient to abdominal exploration. Endoscopy is the first line therapy; in general, if the patient requires more than 4–6 units of blood and the bleeding is not controlled endoscopically, the patient should be managed operatively. Patients who are hemodynamically unstable and have ongoing hemorrhage should also be treated operatively. Other criteria for operative intervention include a rebleeding ulcer that is not controlled by endoscopy and medical therapy and possibly those patients with giant ulcers and a "visible vessel." All patients with endoscopically confirmed peptic ulcers should be given high-dose, intravenous PPI therapy. Also, if the patient tests positive for H. pylori, antibiotic eradication should be initiated and later confirmed.

Operative intervention can be either laparoscopic or open, depending on the surgeon's expertise, severity of bleed, and the localization of the ulcer. For duodenal ulcers, vessel ligation through a longitudinal duodenotomy over the site of the ulcer is performed. Care must be taken to not injure the common bile duct. In contrast, operative treatment for gastric ulcers includes either hemigastrectomy, usually without vagotomy unless it is a distal antral ulcer, or a wedge resection (usually for proximal lesions) with or without proximal gastric vagotomy considering that long-term PPI therapy may be equivalent to proximal vagotomy.

Mortality and re-bleeding after operative treatment of bleeding peptic ulcers is associated with high rates of mortality and re-bleeding.

For these reasons and due to the efficiency of PPI in treatment of peptic ulcer, more recent trends have been to only suture control the bleeding site and to treat the patient aggressively with, postoperative acid suppression as well as medical treatment of any associated H. pylori infection with the drugs now available.

## Variceal Bleeding

Variceal bleeding is responsible for about a third of all cirrhosis-related mortality and must be treated aggressively. Endoscopic hemostasis with band-ligation, injection sclerotherapy, or clip placement is successful in a majority of patients, and the need for emergency porto-systemic shuts has become a treatment of the past. Concomitant drug therapy with octreotide, somatostatin, or glypressin improves bleeding control and outcome(octreotide: 50 mg IV bolus followed by 50 mg per 8-24hrs; Somatostatin: 250-500 mg IV bolus followed by 250-500 mg per hour; Glypressin: 2 mg IV bolus followed by 1mg every 4 hours). If endoscopic control fails, balloon tamponade (Minnesota tube or Sengstaken-Blakemore tube) should be attempted for a maximum 24–48 h followed by endoscopic hemostasis. Once acute bleeding is controlled, treatment with propranolol (40 mg, p.o., b.i.d.) should be initiated; sclerotherapy or band ligation of remaining varices should be performed at weekly intervals until all varices are sclerosed or ligated.

Operative therapy should be avoided whenever possible in patients who are candidates for liver transplantation. If bleeding persists in these patients, a transjugular intrahepatic portosystemic shunt (TIPS) to decompress the portal system is often preferable. This procedure, however, is associated with a mortality of about 10% and hepatic encephalopathy around 20%; therefore, its application is recommended as a bridge to liver transplantation. If bleeding persists or recurs and medical and endoscopic measures fail, then operative intervention is required, but this scenario has become quite uncommon. Patients who are not candidates for liver transplantation and who are stable should undergo a distal splenorenal shunt if the venous anatomy is appropriate; if not, a mesocaval graft, a porto-caval shunt, or a gastric devascularization with esophageal transection is recommended.

## Patients with Schistosomiasis

In patients with portal hypertension secondary to mansonic schistosomiasis, endoscopic sclerosis or rubber banding of bleeding esophageal varices achieve good results in over 90% of patients. Should recurrent bleeding occur, then the operative strategy is to interrupt the left gastric vein and to devascularize the greater curvature of the stomach, and to perform a splenectomy followed by endoscopic sclerosis of esophageal varices.

If varices of the gastric wall are present, it is necessary to oversew the varicose veins through a gastrotomy; treating these specific lesions with endoscopy alone has limited success. Recurrence of bleeding after transgastric ligation of bleeding gastric varices at follow-up of 30 months was 15% and overall mortality was 6%. In portal hypertension due to liver cirrhosis, the approach of azygous-portal disconnection is not considered an adequate procedure, because it is followed by a very high rate of re-bleeding as well as high risk of portal thrombosis.

## Hemorrhagic Gastritis

Severe bleeding from gastritis has become extremely rare. Most bleeding from gastritis is almost always controlled medically with PPIs, $H_2$ receptor blockers, antacids, and/or sucralfate. If medical treatment fails, administration of vasopressin via the left or right gastric arteries should be attempted. In this setting, if medical therapy fails, the results of operative intervention are quite poor, and every attempt should be made to avoid need for operative intervention. If severe bleeding persists, a total or sub-total gastrectomy may be required, however, the need for such an aggressive approach has virtually disappeared. It is for this reason that prophylaxis against stress gastritis for ICU patients with either PPIs or an H2 receptor blocker is recommended. All patients with gastritis should undergo H. pylori screening, and if positive, treatment should be initiated; follow up confirmation of eradication of *H. pylori* is highly recommended.

## Mallory-Weiss Tears

Mallory-Weiss tears result from repeated vomiting. In most patients, the bleeding stops without therapy. If bleeding persists, endoscopic coagulation may be necessary. Only rarely is operative intervention required for direct suture of the tear which can be done through a high anterior gastrotomy.

## Neoplasms

Clinically important, acute bleeding due to neoplasms of the upper GI tract is not common. Some patients with gastric cancer, particularly in early stages, may develop gastric bleeding followed by hematemesis, particularly in patients taking NSAIDs or aspirin. The endoscopic examination should be used to biopsy the lesion to confirm the diagnosis. Usually the bleeding stops spontaneously. Hemorrhage due to advanced gastric cancer that erodes the left gastric artery or another vascular pedicle of the stomach, although rare, may be severe and persistent, making an operative intervention mandatory to resect the tumor or at least to obliterate the bleeding vessel if the malignancy is non-resectable.

Acute bleeding due to an esophageal neoplasm is very rare, although in some instances, advanced carcinoma of the lower third of the esophagus can erode the descending aorta provoking a catastrophic, but terminal hemorrhage.

Gastrointestinal stromal tumors (GIST) may provoke acute bleeding as the first symptom of the disease. The bleeding is usually self-limited, giving time for the diagnosis of site and origin of the blood loss. The treatment is almost always operative, even if palliative, but newer chemotherapeutic options have become available, offering prolonged effective palliation in some of these patients.

Lymphoma is another important cause of bleeding in the GI tract; however, hemorrhage from these lesions usually is not continuous, making the diagnosis and the staging of the disease possible followed by the establishment of a treatment strategy, which is often multidisciplinary.

Adenomas of the upper GI tract, more often located in the small bowel (especially periampullary) but occurring also in the stomach and rarely in the esophagus, may be caused of intense GI bleeding. Treatment may be endoscopic resection or operative.

## Hiatus Hernia and Esophagitis

Esophagitis and hiatus hernia are very rare causes of acute upper GI bleeding as opposed to chronic bleeding; their diagnosis is easily made by endoscopy. Treatment in the acute phase is usually the same as for non-complicated esophagitis and achieves good results in general terms.

## Vascular Lesions

*Dieulafoy lesions*: Dieulafoy's lesion typically presents with intermittent, recurrent, acute upper GI bleeding. The lesion occurs when an abnormally large-caliber submucosal artery becomes exposed at the surface of the mucosa and then ruptures, usually in the stomach, but on occasion in the small bowel. Diagnosis may be quite difficult, even in the stomach, because the lesion is focal and bleeds only intermittently. In contrast, preoperative diagnosis from a lesion in the small bowel requires either endoscopic visualization or demonstration by angiography. Endoscopic methods to treat Dieulafoy's lesion include banding, clipping, electrocautery, cyanoacrylate glue injection, sclerosant injection, epinephrine injection, heat probe, banding, and laser therapy. Angiographic embolization can be tried as well. If these therapies fail, operative control is indicated.

*Aortoenteric fistulas*: Most aortoenteric fistulas occur secondary to erosion into the bowel from a pseudoaneurysm that has formed from the proximal aortic anastomosis after prior placement of an intraabdominal aortic graft; primary aorto-enteric fistulas, although exceedingly rare, can occur from an atherosclerotic or mycotic aortic aneurysm. Most aortoenteric fistulas occur at the level of the distal duodenum or the jejunum and sometimes the colon. These lesions require operative intervention.

*Vascular ectases*: Vascular ectasias or angiodysplasia may be cause of acute GI bleeding but are much more common in the large bowel in older patients. In contrast, small bowel vascular lesions are usually arteriovenous malformations and occur in younger patients <40 years old. When in the stomach or upper part of the duodenum, the hemorrhagic episode may be treated by endoscopic methods. Recently with the development of therapeutic enteroscopes, some patients with bleeding of small bowel arteriovenous malformations have been treated successfully.

# Hemobilia

Loss of blood through biliary tree directly into the duodenal lumen is a very rare condition. Hemobilia is usually secondary to operative trauma, prior percutaneous biliary intubation. The diagnosis is usually made by angiography and treated by arterial embolization. Liver neoplasms may also cause hemobilia.

# Selected Readings

Adler DG, Leighton JA, Davila RE et al. (2004) ASGE guideline: The role of endoscopy in acute non-variceal upper-GI hemorrhage. Gastrointest Endosc 60:497–504

American Gastroenterological Association medical position statement (2000) Evaluation and management of occult and obscure gastrointestinal bleeding. Gastroenterology 118:197–201

Barkun A, Bardou M, Marshall JK (2003) Consensus recommendations for managing patients with nonvariceal upper gastrointestinal bleeding. Ann Intern Med 139:843–857

British Society of Gastroenterology Endoscopy Committee (2002) Nonvariceal upper gastrointestinal haemorrhage: guidelines. Gut 51 (Suppl 4):iv1–6

Esrailian E, Gralnek IM (2005) Nonvariceal upper gastrointestinal bleeding: epidemiology and diagnosis. Gastroenterol Clin North Am 34:589–605

Ferguson CB, Mitchell RM (2005) Nonvariceal upper gastrointestinal bleeding: standard and new treatment. Gastroenterol Clin North Am 34:607–621

Ferraz AAB, Lopes EPA, Barros FMR et al. (2001) Splenectomy + left gastric vein ligature + devascularization of the great curvature of the stomach in the treatment of hepatosplenic schistosomiasis. Postoperative endoscopic sclerosis is necessary? Arq Gastroenterol 38:84–88

Legrand MJ, Jacquet N (1996) Surgical approach in severe bleeding peptic ulcer. Acta Gastroenterol Belg 59:240–244

Manning-Dimmitt LL, Dimmitt SG, Wilson GR (2005) Diagnosis of gastrointestinal bleeding in adults. Am Fam Physician 71:1339–1346

Rockey DC (2005) Occult gastrointestinal bleeding. Gastroenterol Clin North Am 34:699–718

Sava G, Marescaux J, Grevier JF (1980) Place de la vagotomie troncu-laire avec hémostase local dans le traitment de l'ulcere duodénale hémorragique. J Chir (Paris) 117:683–687

Triadafilopoulos G (2005) Review article: the role of anti-secretory therapy in the management of non-variceal upper gastrointestinal bleeding. Aliment Pharmacol Ther 22(Suppl 3):53–58

# Index